# ETHICAL AND MORAL DIMENSIONS OF CARE

# Human Care and Health Series*

### General Editor

**Madeleine M. Leininger,** R.N., M.S.N., Ph.D., L.H.D., D.S., F.A.A.N., C.T.N.
Professor of Nursing and Adjunct Professor of Anthropology
Colleges of Nursing and Liberal Arts
Wayne State University, Detroit

### National Advisory Review Board

**Agnes Aamodt,** R.N., M.S.N., Ph.D.,
F.A.A.N.
Professor of Nursing
College of Nursing
University of Arizona, Tucson

**Delores Gaut,** R.N., M.S.N., Ph.D.
Professor of Nursing
Associate Dean of Graduate Nursing
Program
School of Nursing
University of Colorado, Denver

**Beverly Horn,** R.N., M.S.N., Ph.D.,
C.T.N.
Professor of Nursing
School of Nursing
University of Washington, Seattle

**Patricia Larsen,** R.N., M.S.N.,
D.N.S.
Assistant Professor of Clinical Nursing
University of California, San Francisco

**Marilyn D. Ray,** R.N., M.S.N.,
Ph.D., C.T.N.
Associate Professor of Nursing
Florida Atlantic University
Eminent Scholar of Christine Lynn,
Chair in Nursing, Boca Raton

**Doris Reiman,** R.N., M.S.N., Ph.D.
Professor and Dean of Nursing
University of Texas, Tyler

**Jean Watson,** R.N., M.S.N., Ph.D.,
F.A.A.N.
Professor and Dean of Nursing
School of Nursing
University of Colorado, Denver

*This Series supports selected scholarly papers of the *International Association of
Human Caring*

# ETHICAL AND MORAL DIMENSIONS OF CARE

Edited by
Madeleine M. Leininger, R.N., M.S.N., Ph.D.,
L.H.D., D.S., F.A.A.N., C.T.N.

 WAYNE STATE UNIVERSITY PRESS    DETROIT    1990

**Library of Congress Cataloging-in-Publication Data**

Ethical and moral dimensions of care / edited by Madeleine M.
    Leininger.
            p.      cm. —(Human care and health series)
        Includes bibliographical references.
        ISBN 0-8143-2332-4   :   $19.95
        1. Nursing—Moral and ethical aspects.   2. Nursing ethics.
    I. Leininger, Madeleine M.   II. Series.
    RT85.E77 1990
        174'.2—dc20                                        90-38404
                                                              CIP

This book is dedicated to the many nurses who have deeply valued and practiced care as the essence of nursing, and who have maintained an ethical and moral stance for the health or well-being of those under their professional care. It is dedicated to the creative and committed students, faculty, and clinicians who have forged new lines of thinking and practices to advance the discipline of nursing. In gratitude for the privilege to teach, mentor, and work with many students during the past four decades, I dedicate this book.

The author gratefully acknowledges the contribution of WSU College of Nursing to support the publication of this book.

# Contents

# Preface

In recent years, it has been encouraging to see nurses recognize, value, and systematically study *human care* as the central, unique, and dominant phenomenon that characterizes and explains the discipline of nursing. With this development has come the need for nurses to study the ethical and moral dimensions of human care in order to provide sensitive and knowledgeable care to people. The ethics of care is becoming a major area of study to guide nursing knowledge and decisions. Recently, nurses have had to deal increasingly with ethical care issues related to substance abuse, AIDS, child and elderly abuse, abortion, ethnocentrism, cultural imposition, euthanasia, and other conditions. Nursing ethics or the ethics of care is no longer a phenomenon to be studied and practiced under medical ethics. Nurses who are responsible for human care must discover and establish ethical and moral principles, standards, and guidelines to help them make appropriate judgments and decisions *within* the perspective of nursing.

Another development is multicultural nursing education and service. This means that nurses are expected to know, understand, and function effectively with people from many different cultures, demonstrating sensitivity to and knowledge of differential ethical values and practices. While transcultural nursing has already been established to help nurses learn about care of people from diverse cultures, many nurses have yet to be prepared in transcultural nursing. Shifting nursing's knowledge base from a largely unicultural to a multicultural perspective is a new and major challenge, especially with respect to ethical care. Transcultural knowledge and practice perspectives are essential to help nurses function in our intense multicultural world. Nurse educators, researchers, and practitioners are challenged to study multicultural ethics and moral commitments with new methods of inquiry and different approaches to human care. A major focus is to discover what is similar and different about ethical culture care norms, principles, and standards so that nurses can apply this knowledge to nursing care practices. Currently, there is a real deficit of knowledge about ethical and moral care values among the diverse cultures in the world. Unless nursing focuses on these issues, the knowledge deficit will lead to a crisis, as clients from different cultures and subcultures increase their demands for ethical care nursing judgments and actions that are congruent with their values.

The purpose of this book is to present different issues, perspectives, and research findings bearing on moral and ethical dimensions of human care within a nursing perspective. It is designed to stimulate thinking, develop new lines of inquiry, and generate ethical and moral care knowledge that can be ultimately used to improve client care services. Several expert nurse ethicists, educators, and clinicians involved with the ethics and morality of human care have presented their viewpoints with these goals in mind and have posed a number of unresolved ethical and moral questions. Each chapter should expand the reader's thinking about the ethical and moral aspects of care and should challenge him or her to pursue different lines of inquiry to advance nursing knowledge on the subject.

Some of the papers in this book were originally presented at National Research Care Conferences (established in 1978), and some at the most recent conference, now called the International Association of Human Caring (the name was changed in 1988 to show a worldwide interest in human care). The different scholars' viewpoints generated so much discussion about ethical care that participants urged that these papers be published. The conferences continue to stimulate nurses to explicate the illusive and embedded aspects of human care, and to present their ideas in international forums. An open discovery attitude with a strong caring ethos has been characteristic of these care conferences. Indeed, the annual conferences on human care and the transcultural nursing care conferences (the latter held since 1974) have been the two significant and continuous forums on human care in the field of nursing since the early 1970s. These annual conferences continue to provide new perspectives about human care, which have led to the establishment of a substantive knowledge base about human care as the essence and central domain of nursing. As the initiator and central leader of these two major nursing conferences, I have been most encouraged to see a cadre of nurse scholars, students, and clinicians become excited about and committed to the study of human care and to the use of this knowledge in nursing education and practice. This has been a major development in nursing, and one which has still greater potential to transform nursing. This cultural movement has diffused to other countries where nurse scholars are now focusing on human care.

Human care has become a dominant interest of nurses worldwide and is gradually replacing a preoccupation with medical ethics that is focused on diseases, diagnoses, and symptom identification. The outstanding leadership of nurse care scholars such as Aamodt, Benner, Horn, Gaut, Gadow, Gardner, Leininger, Ray, Reiman, Watson, Thomas, Wenger, and others, have contributed to this worldwide cultural movement to make human care knowledge exciting and meaningful to nurses. Unquestionably, this transcultural care movement can be viewed as one of the most significant developments in the history of nursing, and a focus on ethics of care worldwide has yet to reach its fullest development. Human care research, education, and practice as the central focus of nursing must be fully explicated with ethical aspects and recognized by all nurses in diverse cultures. I predict that human care with a transcultural focus will be nursing's unique discipline contribution to humanity.

This book is the fourth major publication of the "Human Care and Health Series." The three preceding books on human care are *Care: An Essential Human Need* (1981, reprinted in 1988); *Care: The Essence of Nursing and Health* (1984, reprinted in 1988); and *Care: Discovery and Uses in Clinical and Community Nursing* (1988). This fourth book, focused on the ethical and moral dimensions of care, is most timely to address many of the critical issues facing health professionals and consumers worldwide. All four books were reprinted or originally published by Wayne State University Press of Detroit, Michigan, to support the International

Association of Human Caring and the general growing interest of many scholars on the topic of human care. I am most grateful to the contributors of these publications, but especially to the staff of Wayne State University Press including Aimée Ergas for her editorial assistance, Darlene Maxey, and Alice Nigoghosian for their production efforts and for their support and active efforts to make these publications available to many readers. These four care books represent the substantive body of knowledge on the subject of human care in the field of nursing. They offer a sound basis for nursing students and scholars to build upon the work of recognized care scholars and leaders.

Madeleine Leininger

# The Philosophical Foundations of Caring

*Sara T. Fry, R.N., Ph.D., F.A.A.N.*

1

The phenomenon of human caring is analyzed and described. Three models of caring are identified—cultural caring, feminist caring, and humanistic caring. The philosophical foundations of these models are described and their relationships to nursing science and nursing practice are explored. Future study of human caring is encouraged with an emphasis on the use of the models of caring in nursing practice.

The phenomenon of human caring is of interest to many individuals and disciplines. It is often interpreted differently, depending on the disciplinary perspective used in an investigation of caring and on the reasons for studying the caring phenomenon in relationship to specific human conditions or events. Yet all human sciences seem to be interested in human caring, particularly its relationships to gender and roles. Indeed, the fact that this is the eleventh National Research Caring Conference [1989] indicates that the phenomenon of caring is of sustained interest to a number of individuals across the social sciences, the humanities, and the applied sciences.

The phenomenon of human caring is of particular interest to nurses because of the judgments and actions that nurses typically make in patient care. Why are we interested in caring? What is it about caring that captures our attention, our devotion, and our research efforts? What are the moral dimensions of caring, and how might human caring provide a foundation for a distinct nursing ethic?

Answering these questions forces us to analyze the concept of caring, including definitions of the term *caring*, and to systematically examine the phenomenon as it occurs in the literature. The first part of this paper will analyze the concept of caring including the definitions of caring that have appeared over time.

The second part of the paper will focus on several models of caring. Because of the extensive amount of research on the caring phenomenon, it is now possible to recognize several models of caring emerging in the contemporary literature. I have conceptualized these models of caring according to the perspective that they seem to address and have labeled them the cultural model, the feminist model, and the humanistic model. I will briefly describe each model and then focus my attention on the humanistic model of caring. It is interesting to note that several philosophical positions on caring are developing within the last model. These positions have important implications for our understanding of the moral aspects of caring and questions of ethics related to caring behaviors. They also help ground caring as a moral phenomenon within the practice of nursing.

The third part of the paper will raise additional questions that will need to be addressed as current work on the phenomenon of caring and its relations to nursing science and practice evolve.

## Conceptual Dimensions of Caring

The concept of caring appears to have several attributes. First, it is considered a "mode of being in the world," insofar as it is a natural state of human existence and the way that we relate to our world and other human beings (Griffin 1983, 289). This attribute of the concept is especially evident in the work of Martin Heidegger and his metaphysical analysis of being ([1927] 1962). For Heidegger, a fundamental way that humans exist in the world is in "care." He claims: "The totality of Being-in-the-world as a structural whole has revealed itself as care" ([1927] 1962, 274).

This view of care expressed by Heidegger is echoed in the work of Nel Noddings (1984) when she argues for caring as a natural sentiment of being human. Natural caring is neither moral nor nonmoral. It is simply natural—a feeling or an internal sense made universal in the whole species. Natural caring is, in short, one's mode of being (or existence) in the world. It is the type of caring that one commonly sees between a mother and her child, whether human or animal. It is not regarded as moral behavior but rather as natural behavior.

A second attribute of the concept of caring is its status as a precondition for caring behavior. As discussed by Griffin, the concept of caring is a "precondition of caring about things, others, or oneself" (1983, 289). This means that the conceptual *idea* about caring exists as a structural feature of human growth and development before caring behaviors (the process of caring) actually commence.

A third attribute of the concept of caring is its identification with moral and/or social ideals (Griffin 1983, 290). Caring occurs in society in order to serve human needs such as protection from the elements or the need for love. Caring professions exist because they have direct responsibility to build up the best structures that will bring about satisfaction of basic needs. Caring, therefore, is a moral phenomenon associated with the ideals of nursing and the ideals of the community because caring serves the needs of others.

In Griffin's analysis of caring (1983), the meanings of caring are clustered into two main groupings. In one cluster, caring is located along a continuum that begins with terms such as *interest* and *attention* and ends with terms such as *consideration, concern, guidance, protection,* and *serving needs.* Griffin argues that all of these terms are related to what is meant by "taking-care-of" or the activities of the caring phenomenon (Griffin 1983, 290). A second cluster of meanings refers to the attitudes and feelings underlying the activities of caring—attitudes and feelings such as inclination, liking for a person, attachment, desiring to be near someone, and the like.

The two groupings of meaning concern the nonmoral aspects of caring, nonmoral because they do not have characteristics that are widely recognized as belonging to the moral realm. Moral aspects of caring involve human motivations and/or character traits rather than structures and objects, or individual tastes or preferences (Beauchamp 1982, 6). In Griffin's study, moral aspects of caring are characteristics related to the perception of need and the duties to respond to need. Both moral and nonmoral aspects come together to produce the phenomenon of human caring. For example, the nurse perceives the patient's need and engages in several consequent actions that constitute "caring." These actions may involve assessment, recognition of the patient as a person, emotions that energize the caring actions (which may or may not involve such emotions as liking or affection), and certain duties of the nurse. These duties arise out of the interaction between the two human components of the caring relationship, or what Noddings refers to as the "caregiver" and the "one-cared-for" (1984, 19).

The literature on caring frequently contains definitions of these aspects of caring. Leininger defines caring as "those human acts and processes that provide assistance to another individual or group based on an interest in or concern for that human being(s), or to meet an expressed, obvious, or anticipated need" (1984a, 46). Professional care consists of cognitive goals, processes, and acts of professional persons or groups that provide assistance to others to meet obvious or anticipated needs. This definition of caring includes more moral than nonmoral aspects of caring and is particularly directed towaard nurse caring.

Other definitions of caring encompass moral and nonmoral aspects. Gaylin has defined caring as a behavior that is biologically programmed in human nature yet is impaired or reinforced by environmental circumstances (1976, 8). Distinguishing caring from emotions or feelings such as liking, comforting, and wishing well, Mayeroff defines caring as "a process, a way of relating to someone that involves development in time through mutual trust and a deepening and qualitative transformation of the relationship (1971, 1). "To care for another person," he states, "in the most significant sense, is to help him [sic] grow and actualize himself" (1971, 1). These definitions emphasize the moral aspects of caring that are motivations to protect the welfare and maintenance of some person.

Given these attributes of the concept of care and the various definitions of caring in the literature, several models of caring appear to be emerging in the study of the caring phenomenon.

## Models of Caring

At the risk of oversimplifying a very complex web of development in the caring literature, I will group the study of the caring phenomenon into three models. These models are not static or inclusive; yet, they are heuristically important. They demonstrate the development of thought about the caring phenomenon and how the philosphical foundations of caring might influence the future study of caring.

The three models of caring that appear to be emerging from formal and informal study of human caring can be called a cultural model of caring, a feminist model of caring, and a humanistic model of caring. Each model will be described in terms of its primary exemplars. Because the cultural model of caring has a rich historical background, it will be described first.

## Cultural Model of Caring

This model has developed from anthropological and sociological studies of caring behaviors in various world cultures. Leininger defines caring as "an essential human need for the full development, health maintenance, and survival of human beings in all world cultures" (1984a, 3). Based on her research with various cultural groups and the recognition that the caring phenomenon occurs in all of them, Leininger relates care to the survival of the human race. Her research demonstrates how the caring phenomenon has been used universally to reduce intercultural stresses and conflicts and protect human beings throughout the ages. She states:

The anthropologic record of the long survival of humans makes us pause to consider the role of care in the evolution of humankind. Different ecologic, cultural, social, and political contexts have influenced human health care and the survival of the human race. One can speculate that cultures could have destroyed themselves had not humanistic care acts helped to reduce intercultural stresses and conflicts and protect humans [1984a, 5].

Based on knowledge about the nursing role in the health maintenance of individuals, families, and communities, Leininger proposes that transcultural knowledge should be combined with nursing knowledge to guide health interventions and health maintenance in the future. She states:

Transcultural specific and universal care knowledge is greatly needed to guide nursing decisions in caring for individuals, families, and communities. Such knowledge would be essentially new and would provide rich bases for guiding nursing education and practice. Knowledge of all cultures will someday be a major and powerful course supporting nursing principles and the laws that guide nurses' thoughts and actions. That day is in the distant future [1984a, 7].

Central to this model is the view that humanistic and scientific caring behaviors, values, and expressions exist in all human cultures, but they are expressed differently and are often covert. Study is required to systematically uncover the caring phenomenon in all cultures and to relate the caring phenomenon to health. Some research on cultural aspects of caring and health has been conducted by past participants of the caring conferences. Examples include Boyle's study of the indigenous caring practices in a Guatemalan colony (1984); Leininger's study of southern rural Afro-American and Anglo-American cultures with a focus on care, health values, beliefs, and practices (1984b); and Dugan's study of caring behaviors (especially social allegiance) among urban Latin groups (1984).

Each of these studies used cultural knowledge and nursing knowledge to elucidate the caring behaviors practiced in these groups. The behaviors were considered reflective of cultural perspectives related to health. As Boyle concluded in her study: "The self and family care activities and associate belief systems described . . . reflect a culturally based body of knowledge that contains the underlying rationales of actions taken to promote health and prevent illness. . . . This shared knowledge is used in purposive action, since the behaviors instigated by sample members to avoid illness, for the most part, follow directly from identified concepts" (1984, 131–32).

Other studies within the cultural model of caring have focused on groups formed for specific purposes that develop a culture derived from the purpose of the group and the participants in the group. A good example is Ray's studies of institutional caring (1984), as well as Wang's studies of Appalachian clinics and the types of caretaker-child interactions observed in the clinic settings (1984). Both of these studies use anthropological methods of investigation and focus on the cultural aspects of group and individual behaviors.

The cultural model of caring appears to be well established in the literature. Additional studies continually expand on the cultural aspects of caring. Indeed, the knowledge gained from studies conducted within this model is usually referred to as transcultural, and the application of this knowledge to the practice of nursing is called transcultural nursing. A central tenet of transcultural nursing is that caring is the essence of professional nursing and that systematic study of the caring phenomenon will characterize nursing with its uniqueness and central purpose. As Leininger claims, the science of nursing practice is the science of caring (1984a) with humanistic perspectives.

## Feminist Model of Caring

A second model in the literature is the feminist model of caring. The work of Nel Noddings (1984) exemplifies this model, although others' versions of the model can also be found in the social science and philosophical literature.

Essentially, this model is theoretically based on ethics and social psychology. Building on the work of Carol Gilligan (1977, 1979, 1982), Noddings, for example has combined knowledge of ethics with a feminist perspective on moral development. She states her purpose and the foundations of her views in the following manner:

> [E]thical argumentation has frequently proceeded as if it were governed by the logical necessity characteristic of geometry. It has concentrated on the establishment of principles and that which can be logically derived from them. One might say that ethics has been discussed largely in the language of the father: in principles and propositions, in terms such as justification, fairness, justice. The mother's voice has been silent. Human caring and the memory of caring and being cared for, which I shall argue form the foundation of ethical response, have not received attention except as outcomes of ethical behavior. . . . I suggest the approach of the mother . . . a feminine view . . . feminine in the deep classical sense, rooted in receptivity, relatedness, and responsiveness. . . . It may be the case that such an approach is more typical of women than of men [1984, 1–2].

A systematic analysis of gender related to transcultural caring behaviors is not addressed by Noddings. In fact, some of the central elements of caring developed within the cultural model are entirely missing in Nodding's version of the feminist model of caring. For example, the relation of caring behaviors to health practices and maintenance is not addressed. However, Noddings does describe how one comes to possess caring behaviors and how caring is expressed in significant human relationships, in general.

Although Noddings is careful to point out that her view of caring is both feminine and masculine, she tends to conflate certain types of ethical positions with gender: to think in terms of ethical principles and rules is masculine; to think in terms of feelings, needs, impressions, and personal ideals is feminine. While she describes the caring phenomenon, in general, as an attitude, she claims that feminine caring expresses our earliest memories of being cared for. In this sense, one's store of memories of both caring and being cared for is always universally accessible but seems necessarily linked to the female figure.

One purpose of Noddings's feminist model of caring is to establish a comprehensive view of caring that is related to ethical behavior and choices. Rather than a model of caring, Noddings's approach could even be considered a model of ethics that simply uses caring as a central component. This is very evident in her definition of care. She states, "to care may mean to be charged with the protection, welfare, or maintenance of something or someone" (1984, 9). In other words, to care is to engage in certain behaviors that have ethical dimensions.

Developing her idea of care further, Noddings focuses on the caring behaviors of human interaction, recognizing that caring behaviors can, and often do, have moral content. The caring behaviors that she describes are the behaviors of receptivity, relatedness, and responsiveness—behaviors that are inherently feminine, she claims, but which can be adopted or embraced by men, even though it is not within their nature to adopt such notions.

Unlike the cultural model of caring, which has tremendous implications for nursing practice, the feminist model of caring has greater implications for education. Basing her analysis of caring on practical ethics, Noddings sees the logical outcome of her study to be revisions in moral education. She describes these implications in the following manner:

"From the view we have taken (the caring phenomenon), such a discussion (of moral education) is of vital importance, for we all bear a responsibility for the ethical perfection of others. Moral education is, then, a community-wide enterprise and not a task exclusively reserved for home, church, or school. . . . [I]t refers to an education that will enhance the ethical ideal of those being educated so that they will continue to meet others morally," (1984, 171).

Scholarship on the caring phenomenon, in general, has been strongly influenced by the feminist model. It has stressed the ethics and morality of caring from a viewpoint that is, despite Noddings's claims to the contrary, gender related. Yet, the model's relevance to nursing knowledge, in general, remains unexplored. Within nursing ethics, however, I suspect that those who recognize the limitations of the biomedical model of ethics may find the feminine model a rich ground for the future discussion of the nursing ethic and for further descriptive study of ethical judgments made by nurses.

## Humanistic Model of Caring

The humanistic model of caring is one of the most interesting model and seems to have three distinct versions. One version has been developed by Jean Watson

(1985) in her work on humanistic nursing theory. Another version has been described by Edmund Pellegrino (1985), a physician and a humanist. A third version can be found in the writings of William Frankena, a philosopher (1983). I will briefly describe each of these versions of the model.

*Watson's Human Caring.* This version of the humanistic model of caring contains several assumptions about human caring, the practice of nursing, and the development of nursing as a science. Its philosophical foundation are found in statements claiming that "caring calls for a philosophy of moral commitment toward protecting human dignity and preserving humanity" (Watson 1985, 31). For Watson, caring is a value and an attitude that has to become a will, an intention, or a commitment that "manifests itself in concrete acts" (1985, 32).

According to Watson, caring is also an ideal that transcends the set of caring in order to influence collective acts of the nursing profession, with important implications for human civilization. Thus, for Watson, human caring eventually becomes a philosophy of action to meet individual needs and to assist the welfare of others. This philosophy is laced with many metaphysical notions of humans and their environment, which undoubtedly enrich the moral context for human caring.

There are very close connections between Watson's and Noddings's views of human caring. Noddings, however, constructs a feminist view of caring, while Watson constructs a general view of caring related to nursing science that is neither male nor female. Watson's view is simply related to a function of nursing (caring) and a basic human need for caring, neither of which is gender related. It is possible that Watson's view of caring could include Noddings's feminine perspective but this would certainly limit the scope of her model. I suspect that Watson would not find this limitation desirable for her conception of caring and its role in nursing science.

*Pellegrino's Moral-Obligation Caring.* Discussing the relationship between the physician and the patient, Pellegrino notes that there are at least four senses in which the word *care* is understood by the health professions. The first sense is "care as compassion" or being concerned for another person (1985, 10). This is a feeling, a sharing of someone's experience of illness and pain, or just being touched by the plight of another person. To care in this sense, according to Pellegrino, is "to see the person who is ill" as more than the object of our ministrations (1985, 11). He or she is "a fellow human whose experiences we cannot penetrate fully but which we can be touched by simply because we share the same humanity" (1985, 11).

*advocacy*

The second sense of caring is "doing for others" what they cannot do for themselves (1985, 11). This entails assisting others with the activities of daily living that are compromised by illness (feeding, bathing, clothing, meeting personal needs). Pellegrino recognizes that physicians do little of this type of caring but that nurses do a great deal. However, nurses do far less of this type of caring than they used to do. According to Pellegrino, nurses' aides do most of this type of caring in contemporary versions of team nursing (1984, 12).

Pellegrino's third sense of caring is caring for the medical problem experienced by the patient. It includes inviting the patient to transfer responsibility and anxiety about what is wrong to the doctor or the nurse. It is a type of caring that ensures

*19*

that knowledge and skill will be directed to the patient's problem. It also recognizes that the patient's anxiety needs a specialized type of caring.

Pellegrino's fourth sense of caring is to *take care* (1985, 12). This entails carrying out all the necessary procedures (personal and technical) in patient care with conscientious attention. Pellegrino claims that this sense of caring is a corollary to the third sense, but argues that it is differentiated by its emphasis on the craftsmanship of medicine. Together, the third and fourth senses of caring constitute what most physicians understand as *competence.*

For Pellegrino, these four senses of caring are not separable in clinical practice. Care that includes the four senses of caring is called "integral care" and is a moral obligation of health professionals (1985, 13). Such caring is not an option that can be exercised or interpreted "in terms of some idiosyncratic definition of professional responsibility," argues Pellegrino (1985, 13). The moral obligation to care in this manner is created by the special human relationship that brings together the one who is ill and the one who offers to help.

In assessing whether the curing or caring models are foundational for clinical practice, Pellegrino reexamines the roles of physicians to their patients. He concludes that "to care for the patient in the full and integral sense, requires a reconstruction of medical ethics" (1985, 17). What is needed is an ethic that recognizes caring as a strong moral obligation between patient and professional.

Central to Pellegrino's ethic of care is the good of the individual, a compounded notion that has at least three components. He states, "a morally good clinical decision should attend to all three senses of patient good and satisfactorily resolve conflicts among them" (1985, 20). The first sense of good is "biomedical good"—the good medical intervention can offer by modifying the natural history of disease in a patient. It uses the craftsmanship of physicians and nurses, the knowledge of science, and indications for treatment (1985, 21). The second sense of good is the patient's concept of his or her own good. It takes into consideration what the patient thinks is worthwhile or in his or her best interests, and can be delegated to a surrogate decision maker (1985, 21). The third sense of patient good is "the good most proper to being human" (1985, 22). For Pellegrino, this is the capacity to make choices, to set up a life plan, and to determine one's goals for a satisfactory life. It fulfills our potentialities as rational indivduals and expresses human freedom and dignity.

Pellegrino contrasts these three senses of patient good with each other and societal ideas of social good. He argues that patient good comes before any other notion of good. Patient good is what ultimately guides decision making in the caring, curing, and coping aspects of treatment for health and illness states (1985, 22). Pellegrino's account of care is similar to both Watson's and Noddings's views. His notion of care is strongly linked to moral conduct between persons. However, it does not include the gender specifications that are present in Noddings's work and does not seem to view physician and nurse caring differently except in intensity and degree. Nonetheless, his model of caring fits the practical sense of nursing science. It also seems to include the notion of human caring that is peculiar to cultural caring.

*Frankena's Moral-Point-of-View Toward Caring.* The final version of the humanistic model of caring is the moral-point-of-view (MPV) version. It is discussed by William Frankena, a well-known MPV theorist, in his critique of other MPV theories (MPVT) (1983).

The term *moral-point-of-view* appeared in the philosophical literature during the early 1950s and was subsequently popularized by philosopher Kurt Baier's book *Taking the Moral Point of View* (1965). The term, however, was a prominent heading in Hegel's *Phenomenology of Mind* ([1807] 1967) and was discussed in the work of Hume ([1751] 1957), Kant ([1785] 1964), and others. The MPV is associated with a certain type of ethical theory of which Frankena seems to be a major spokesman.

One takes an MPV by (a) subscribing to a particular substantive moral principle, (b) taking a general approach, perspective, stance, or vantage point from which to proceed (which occurs whenever anyone makes judgments of certain sorts), and (c) by adopting a general outlook or method appropriate to reaching conclusions in a particular field of inquiry (Frankena, 1983). An MPVT is a meta-ethical or metamoral theory. Such a theory contains views about moral judgments and principles, about the differences between them and nonmoral principles, and about the general nature of their justification. It may not entail subscribing to any principle, but "it may entail believing that the MPV should be defined in a certain way" (Frankena 1983, 41). Such theories tend to do four things (not necessarily jointly): (a) define morality or the distinction between the moral and the nonmoral, (b) formulate and establish a test for determining which moral judgments and norms are true, valid, or justified, (c) analyze what animates morality or makes it tick, (d) attempt to show why we should be moral. In short, an MPVT insists that we "take the MPV explicitly or implicitly, in arriving at our most basic moral judgments, whatever these are, at least when we make them first-hand" (Frankena 1983, 43).

For Baier, taking the MPV means to adopt a certain point by defining its principle. In other words, one takes the MPV by stating the "marks of the moral" or the criteria for moral judgments (for example, universality, prescriptiveness, overriding authority, and reference to the welfare of others) (Baier 1965, 101). Others, including Frankena, have tended to take the MPV differently than Baier. Taylor, for example, argues that taking the MPV is to decide the appropriate rules of relevance for a moral stance. In an often-quoted article, "On Taking the Moral Point of View" (1978, 36), Taylor gives his own version of the marks of the moral according to features present in Western morality (generality, universality, overriding nature, disinterestedness, publicness, and impartiality).

In addition to the views of Baier and Taylor, Frankena reviews other MPVTs and notes the principles that are central to the particular MPVT. For example, sympathy was a major principle in Hume's theory; agape has been a central principle in Christian theories. He then offers his own principle, which he claims is more neutral than benevolence, love, or sympathy. Frankena's principle for taking the moral-point-of view is caring about persons. He states: "I have suggested that taking the MPV is or includes a kind of direct Caring about or Non-Indifference to what goes on in the lives of people and consciously sentient beings as such, including others besides oneself. . . . [I]t includes not only making normative judgments but making nonhypothetical ones as well" (1983, 74–75).

What is caring for Frankena? "Caring need not take the form of love," he states, "it may simply take the more Kantian form of respect for persons. . . . It is "the attitude" of attributing 'intrinsic worth' to persons or conscious sentient beings" (1983, 75). Frankena's principle of caring means to respect persons as well as to offer individuals unconditional love.

Frankena's view of caring is vastly different from Noddings's view of caring. It includes the notion of duty but clearly does not include the notion of reciprocal caring important to the feminist model. For much of moral philosophy, taking the moral-point-of-view is simply acting on principle or out of duty, and requires no response from the one who is cared for to the one who cares.

Frankena's view of caring is also different from Noddings's view in that caring as a principle of nonindifference is neither male nor female. Where Noddings argues that caring is primarily a female tendency, Frankena's caring is easily adopted by both males and females. To respect persons is to respect human dignity, not female or male gender.

However, Frankena's version of the humanistic model of caring helps us to see that many of the caring models are, in fact, adopting a moral-point-of-view. This is certainly the case with Watson, Pellegrino, Noddings, and Frankena. His model also helps us to see the important implications of a humanistic model of caring and the relevance of ethical analysis to the caring phenomenon.

## Conclusions

All three of the models of caring have important implications for nursing research and the future development of theories of caring. Yet, at least three sets of questions need to be addressed before additional work on the caring phenomenon in nursing proceeds. First, what is the relation between ethical inquiry, discussions on morality, and caring research? Is all caring work necessarily also ethics? Given the current scope of inquiry on the caring phenomenon, this does not seem likely. Inquiry on the caring phenomenon can be social, anthropological, psychological, or ethical in nature.

Second, does a model of caring in nursing necessarily have to be gender related? In other words, is it more desirable to have a feminist model of caring for nursing than any other model? Or, is the nature of the caring phenomenon such that one does not need to regard caring as either masculine or feminine *or* as related to the gender dominance of a professional practice?

Third, can humanistic and and anthropological models of caring exist side by side without one necessarily attempting to cover the ground of the other? It is reasonable to think that they can. An anthropological view of caring will resort to anthropological theories and cultural components that are not necessarily important to a humanistic model of caring. Likewise, a humanistic model of caring need not address the cultural dimensions of caring. The basis for a humanistic model of caring will understandably be moral values. In such a model, caring is an existential phenomenon that can be viewed in its moral context as opposed to its cultural context. While the anthropologist will primarily be interested in the cultural aspects of caring, philosophers and others will be interested in the humanistic aspects of caring.

As a final point, it will be important for any research efforts to define, expand, and even juxtapose alternatives to the caring models presented here. As this occurs, we should anticipate that research will more adequately address the potential uses of models of care and enlarge our understanding of the caring phenomenon in human existence.

# References

Baier, K. 1965. *The moral point of view: A rational basis of ethics.* New York: Random House.

Beauchamp, T. L. 1982. *Philosophical ethics.* New York: McGraw-Hill.

Boyle, J. 1984. Indigenous caring practices in a Guatemalan colonia. In *Care: The essence of nursing and health,* edited by M. Leininger, 123–32. Thorofare, NJ: Charles B. Slack.

Dugan, A.B. 1984. Compadrazgo: A caring phenomenon among urban Latinos and its relationship to health. In *Care: The essence of nursing and health,* edited by M. Leininger, 183–94. Thorofare, NJ: Charles B. Slack.

Frankena, W. K. 1983. Moral-point-of-view theories. Ini *Ethical theory in the last quarter of the twentieth century,* edited by N. E. Bowie, 39–79. Indianapolis: Hackett.

Gaylin, W. 1976. *Caring.* New York: Avon Books.

Gilligan, C. 1977. In a different voice: Women's conception of self and of morality. *Harvard Educational Review* 47: 481–517.

Gilligan, C. 1979. Woman's place in man's life cycle. *Harvard Educational Review* 49: 431–46.

Gilligan, C. 1982. *In a different voice: Psychological theory and women's development.* Cambridge: Harvard University Press.

Griffin, A.P. 1983. A philosophical analysis of caring in nursing. *Journal of Advanced Nursing* 8: 289–95.

Hegel, G. W. F. (1807) 1967. *The phenomenology of mind,* translated by J. B. Baillie. New York: Harper & Row.

Heidegger, M. (1927) 1962. *Being and time,* translated by J. Macquarrie and E. Robinson. New York: Harper & Row.

Hume, D. (1751) 1957. *An inquiry concerning the principles of morals.* Indianapolis: Bobbs-Merrill.

Kant, I. (1785) 1964. *Groundwork of the metaphysics of morals,* translated by H. J. Paton. New York: Harper & Row.

Leininger, M.M. 1981. *Caring: An essential human need. Proceedings of the Three National Caring Conferences.* Thorofare, NJ: Charles B. Slack.

Leininger, M. M. 1984a. *Care: The essence of nursing and health.* Thorofare, NJ: Charles B. Slack.

Leininger, M. M. 1984b. Southern rural black & white American lifeways with focus on care & health phenomena. In *Care: The essence of nursing and health,* 133–59). Thorofare, NJ: Charles B. Slack.

Mayeroff, M. 1971. *On caring.* New York: Harper & Row.

Noddings, N. 1984. *Caring: A feminine approach to ethics and moral education.* Berkeley: University of California Press.

Pellegrino, E. 1985. The caring ethic: The relation of physician to patient. In *Caring, curing, coping: Nurse, physician, patient relationships,* edited by A. H. Bishop & J. R. Scudder, 8–30. University, AL: University of Alabama Press.

Ray, M.A. 1984. The development of a classification system of caring. In *Care: The essence of nursing and health,* edited by M. M. Leininger, 95–112. Thorofare, NJ: Slack.

Taylor, P.W. 1978. On taking the moral point of view. *Midwest Studies in Philosophy* III:35–61.

Wang, J. F. 1984. Caretaker-child interaction observed in two Appalachian clinics. In *Care: The essence of nursing and health,* edited by M. M. Leininger, 195–215). Thorofare, NJ: Slack.

Watson, J. 1985. *Nursing: Human science and human care. A theory of nursing.* Norwalk, CT: Appleton-Century-Crofts.

# Are There Limits to Caring?:
# Conflict Between Autonomy and Beneficence

*Anne J. Davis, R.N., Ph.D., F.A.A.N.*

2

The dominant theme of this paper is the conflict between autonomy and beneficence in ethical care and related professional services. The author argues that neither moral principles and absolutes nor the ethics of natural caring can act as sufficient guidelines for a moral life or in decision making. Instead these dimensions need to be considered together to deal with ethical dilemmas and possible solutions in any given situation. Several ethical and moral dilemmas are presented to substantiate conflicts between autonomy and beneficence in professional caring. The importance of respect for persons is a critical ethical principle in caring for or caring about patients, which is best realized in an environment of caring for the caregivers.

In her book *Caring: A Feminine Approach to Ethics and Moral Education*, Nel Noddings says:

We want to be moral in order to remain in the caring relation and to enhance the ideal of ourselves as one caring. . . . Everything depends upon the nature and strength of this ideal, for we shall not have absolute principles to guide us. Indeed, I shall reject ethics of principle as ambiguous and unstable. Wherever there is a principle, there is implied its exception and, too often, principles function to separate us from each other (1984, 5).

However, a few pages later she also says that the ethics of caring has limits. Specifically, "another sort of conflict occurs when what the cared-for wants is not what we think would be best for him" (1984, 5). In such a situation as this, what do we look to as guidelines in an attempt to be ethical?

Most individuals who have given much thought to it would agree that the ethics of principles is limited and without absolutes to guide us. Additionally, anyone who has thought about this further might say that the notion of absolutes enacted in the everyday world, taken seriously and literally, might become what one philosopher calls the tyranny of principles. If the cult of absolute principles is so attractive today, it means that we still find it impossible to break with the "quest for certainty" that John Dewey tried so hard to discredit (Toulmin 1987).

But let me remind you that Dewey was not the first to point out the shortcomings of absolutism. Aristotle himself insisted that there are no *essences* in the realm of ethics. Practical reasoning in ethics, as elsewhere, is a matter of judgment, of weighing different considerations against one another, and never a matter of formal theoretical deduction from strict or self-evident axioms. It is a task less for the clever arguer than for the large-spirited human being (Aristotle 1962). I am not convinced that the ethics of caring gives us absolutes either, assuming they are both good and necessary as Noddings seems to.

Moral enthusiasts who assume absolutes and try to impose rigid rules set the stage for abuse. History enlightens us about absolutism as it points to both the Jesuit casuists and Talmudic scholars, who while being human and imperfect, did grasp the essential Aristotelian idea that practical ethics and the large-spirited human attitude help us to travel the complex territory of the moral life and moral problems. I would argue that neither the anemic portrayal of ethics as merely principles and absolutes nor the ethics of natural caring can act as sufficient guidelines for a moral life. Both are limited, and the question is whether together they can help us gain insights into, and sensitivity regarding, the ethical dilemmas confronting us and to possible solutions to find a given situation.

While I think of myself as a feminist, I find it difficult to embrace natural caring without the benefit of the additional assistance I received from ethical principles and ethical reasoning. While I realize that I have no absolutes from the latter, I view this as desirable because it demands that I call into play my ability *to care* and *to think*. Both of these behaviors help to move me toward the ideal: the development of myself as a large-spirited human being. What Aristotle discussed was, of course, the virtuous and not ethical principles.

As regards the virtues, let me turn to McIntyre (1981), who uses the Aristotelian tradition in two distinct places in his argument. He suggests that a great part of modern morality is intelligible only as a set of surviving fragments from that tradition. Indeed he goes on to say that the inability of modern moral philosophers to carry through their projects of analysis and justification is closely connected with the fact that the concepts with which they work are a combination of surviving fragments and implausible modern inventions. But in addition to this, the rejection of the Aristotelian tradition was one in which ethical rules and principles, so predominant in modern conceptions of morality, become the focus and ingredients of moral reasoning, removing the virtues from their central place.

Moral philosophers list principles in different order, depending on which they define as root principles. These principles can assist us in determining what is a right or wrong action and can serve in decision making. Two philosophers, Downie and Telfer (1970), have indicated that the one basic principle is respect for persons and that all other principles emerge from this one. But to be respectful of persons requires an attitude of caring and seems to be more akin to the idea of moral character or virtue. As Aristotle said, virtues are habits or traits of character that predispose one to do what is right (Aristotle 1962). According to Fowler (1986), perhaps the best way to think of the ethics of caring and the ethics of principles is to realize that virtues grounded in caring and duties grounded in ethical principles should be thought of as inseparable, for the norms of obligation without corresponding character traits are useless; character traits without norms of obligation are directionless (1986, 528–530).

The above discusssion has not dealt with the fact that even within the relatively coherent tradition of Western ethical thought, there are many different and incompatible conceptions of virtue. With this in mind, I now turn to a specific ethical dilemma that often confronts health professionals. This dilemma emerges in those situations where the patient's autonomy and the caregiver's obligation to do no harm may conflict. This presents us with one of the noted limitations in the ethics of caring. Noddings referred to this dilemma when she said, "another sort of conflict occurs when what the cared-for wants is not what we think would be best for him [sic]" (1984, 5).

A philosophical theme found in the Western tradition is that the essence of tragedy is the conflict of one good with another. This papers focuses on such a situation: when the patient's autonomy and the health care professional's obligation conflict. While I will focus on notions of rights and obligations, such a focus is to be understood within the context of caring. As I have written elsewhere, one meaning of *caring* is to suffer with, to undergo with, to share solidarity with. This meaning moves us away from the more limited definition implied in the phrases *nursing care* or *medical care*, where caring often means the use of technical knowledge and skill, but does not necessarily include caring as an attitude toward the patient. Professional socialization, role models, and the dominant value system of cure and efficiency in hospitals can limit caring to technical knowledge and skill, whereas situations often call for an unfolding of our most basic human qualities to the other person. The most demanding and deeply human aspect of caring is the art of being fully present to another; it is both caring for and caring about (Davis 1981).

Lucy Van Pelt of *Peanuts* fame once said that she could love humanity, it was just people she could not tolerate. I take this statement to mean that it is easier to speak in the great abstract than it is sometimes to deal with situations in everyday life. This could apply to a situation in which the patient's autonomy and the health professional's obligation conflict. And while an attitude and an ethics of caring are important in order to have a caring environment within which to think about and work through this ethical dilemma, by themselves this attitude and this ethic will not tell us what we should do. But since we have no absolutes in ethical principles, how are we to think about this dilemma? Let us examine these principles more fully.

## Autonomy

In the western philosophical tradition, autonomy stands as a central concept. While it has less potency outside that tradition, it must be examined within that context. Autonomy, the self-directed capacity to determine and carry out one's life plan, contains two features: independence and totality (Jassi 1977). Independence is the ability to take responsibility for one's life by acting on the surrounding influences. Action is taken according to some overall plan, and it results in life displaying a totality. Autonomy is associated with a "family of ideas": freedom of choice, choosing for oneself, creating one's own moral position, and accepting responsibility for one's moral views. The capacity for autonomy is considered inherent in all persons, yet the principle of autonomy applies only to the individual capable of autonomous action. The first perspective of autonomy as requiring some rational evaluation and decision-making ability assumes the individual is competent (Beauchamp and Childress

1983). Many patients are competent to make their own decisions provided that they are given enough information that they can understand. This occurs, of necessity, within a context of caring. Informed consent says that we give the information that a reasonable person would want, plus what the individual wants to know. This allows persons to make their own decisions.

There are several interesting notions that need to be mentioned here. First, competency is sometimes in the eye of the beholder. That is, provided you, the patient, make the decision that I, the health professional, think you ought to make, you are competent in my opinion. This is one of the bases of the potential conflict. When people do have the right and opportunity to make decisions, they can and sometimes do make the "wrong" decision. Here we must relinquish the notion of "wrong." What would have to occur for a person's decision about himself or herself to be considered wrong? Such a decision could be based on insufficient quantity or quality of information, or the patient's refusal to accept the information as untainted or true. Another example of a "wrong" decision occurs when the patient cannot fully appreciate the risks and benefits involved in a treatment because the threat of pain cannot be balanced against the risks of the treatment with clear judgment. The concept of autonomy helps to establish moral independence. Not only does it entail that I, as an autonomous individual, am to be treated by others as a moral end rather than as a moral means, but it also requires that they allow me to pursue my own moral goods.

The moral autonomy of others does not rule out attempts to persuade them to think or act differently. What we should not do is impose our values or the dictates of our conscience on them against their will. While autonomy is a moral good, it is not a moral obsession. Autonomy pushed to the outer limits means we have no such thing as a common good since we are left with only the aggregate of individual goods (Callahan 1984).

Let me be more specific and limit my comments to the clinical and moral dilemma of a patient refusing lifesaving treatment. Although there is a right to autonomy that ethically justifies patients refusing lifesaving treatment, this right is not absolute, since medical judgment can override it under certain limited circumstances. While some seek absolutes, it seems to me that they are not possible, not necessary, and not even a good idea, morally speaking. Acknowledging the limits of patient autonomy does not mean that the latter can be overriden when it comes into conflict with the judgments of health care professionals. It is not a situation of all or nothing; that is, we do not say that in all cases autonomy is given moral priority, and we do not say that in all cases autonomy is overriden. Life is too complex for this approach.

One way around this possible impasse between autonomy as the moral priority and the problem of overriding autonomy is to make a list of variables that would have to be taken into account if the refusal of lifesaving treatment should be suspected. Such a list would include life expectancy with and without treatment, age, extent of pain and suffering, views of those in the situation, and cost. Such a list, however, is not without problems. First, one could add or substract different variables and always override autonomy; and second, this approach shifts the focus of our concern from the patient's refusal to the patient's condition and demographic data. This means that the decision is *about* the patient, not *by* the patient (Miller 1981).

One helpful way of thinking about autonomy is to realize that our usual definitions of self-determination (the right to make one's own decisions) and respect for autonomy (the obligation not to interfere with another's choice and to treat the other as capable of choosing) gives us only a bare-bones definition. We need more than this definition for the analysis of any given situation. Miller has given us four senses of this concept as it is used in bioethics. Briefly, they are: (a) autonomy as free action, which means that an action is voluntary and intentional rather than the result of coercion, duress, or undue influence; (b) autonomy as authenticity, which means that an action is consistent with the person's attitudes, values, dispositions, and life plans; we say the person is acting in character; (c) autonomy as effective deliberation or actions taken, where a person believes that he or she is in a situation calling for a decision, is aware of the alternatives and the consequences of those alternatives, can evaluate both, and can choose an action based on that evaluation; and finally, (d) autonomy as moral reflection, which means acceptance of the moral values one acts on. This requires rigorous self-analysis because we so often engage in piecemeal or occasional moral reflection. All of this requires more moral reflection on the part of all of us, whether patient or health professional (Miller 1981).

## Beneficence

Beneficence, or doing good, is difficult to discuss without taking into account another ethical principle namely, nonmaleficence, which means an obligation to do no harm. Indeed, some philosophers do not separate these principles from one another. Others, however, do separate them and go on to say that health professionals have a greater duty to do no harm than they have to do good. The interesting question here is, What constitutes harm and what constitutes doing good? And when I raise the question in this fashion, I imply that some definitions of doing good can also be viewed as possibly doing harm. This implies that there is more than one way to conceptualize the notion of harm. Often in the health care arena we tend to limit our notions of harm to physical harm. But there are other kinds of harms as well, such as psychological harm, social harm, and ethical harm, in the sense of treating people as merely means, or of not respecting them as persons.

There are times when the limited definition of harm is tied to the notion of a situation needing a "merely medical" solution, as if such a solution in itself is value free or that it can be considered in an ethical vacuum. In addition, this basic problem can be compounded by the health professional's use of a central concept: patient need. Again, need is often defined merely as medical need. Doing good has been primarily thought of as meeting the patient's needs and acting to decrease or resolve them. Both of these concepts, "merely medical" and "patient need," can lend themselves to paternalistic actions on the part of health professionals. However, one need often attributed to adults is their ability to act as competent, autonomous persons and to make decisions that have an impact on their health care and well-being.

Can health care professionals actually cause harm and fail in their duty to do no harm by attempting to meet patients' needs regardless of whether their actions are paternalistic? The basic question here is, Do some types of caring have within them the potential seeds of harm? There is a provocative line in the film *Sunday Bloody Sunday* (1971, directed by John Schlesinger) in which Glenda Jackson says: "There are times when nothing is better than something."

The principle of double effects helps us to think about this problem. We can think both of harm from meeting needs in certain instances and of those situations where needs go unmet. The principle of double effects is based on four conditions: (a) the action in itself must be good or at least morally indifferent, (b) the agent must intend only the good effect and not the evil effect, (c) the evil effect cannot be a means to the good effect, and (d) there must be a proportionality between the benefits and burdens of the action (Beauchamp and Childress 1983). While such a principle does not give us absolutes, it can help us pose the ethical dilemma and work toward a solution.

In general, given the situation of a patient refusing lifesaving treatment, we could reason as follows: The actions of meeting people's needs is good according to the duty of beneficence. Providers intend only good effects. In cases in which the patient's autonomy must be infringed upon to do good, the evil of overriding autonomy becomes a means to this good. Such infringement on individual autonomy, even to meet a patient's needs, is difficult to justify ethically. Consideration of each individual would be based on proportionality between good and evil effects of the intervention. The principle of double effects does provide justification for the side effects of unmet needs if rights are promoted (Garritson and Davis 1983). This does not negate the earlier position that not always are rights absolute. We must take into account the four-dimensional definition of autonomy developed by Miller, which I mentioned earlier. As Callahan (1984) said, autonomy is a moral good and not a moral obsession. These more complex senses of autonomy and this thinking about professional ethical obligations toward patients give us some general guidelines as to what we should do. To ask for moral absolutes from any source seems unreasonable and possibly even dangerous. When we use principle-based ethical reasoning or when we use ethics of caring, we must first ground our concern and questioning in the concreteness of a given situation.

In undertaking clinical ethics consultation in hospitals focused on the question of withdrawing treatment or patient refusal of treatment, I use ethical principles, an attitude of caring, and as much information about the patient situation as possible. To do otherwise is to act as if I had absolutes. When asking about the patient, the questions become: Who is this human being? What does he or she hold to be valuable and true? Questions concerning the diagnosis and prognosis are important, but serve merely to create the backdrop against which questions of human values are discussed. From this vantage point, I am not convinced that there is such as thing as "merely medical," but I am convinced that there are limits to caring.

As a health professional, I can give care to and I can care about another. While these notions of caring are not mutually exclusive, caring about is the more deeply ethical sensitivity and provides the humane context in which caring for or giving care to occurs. A health professional's zeal to meet ethical obligations in giving care to or caring for may conflict with this larger sense of caring, which in some circumstances may mean more caring about and less care for, especially when we define *care for* as treatment. I would argue that medical treatment and nursing care are different, but that is another matter.

A clinical nurse once came to me and said that the nurses in a critical care unit wanted to act as a patient advocate. They wanted to form a committee of nurses to review all research protocols and decide which of the patients would or would not be allowed to be approached for informed consent. After I asked about the patients and was told that they were able to give consent, I asked why such a committee of nurses was necessary. The answer essentially was that these nurses cared for the patients and believed that they had an obligation to safeguard them from harm. Thus, a committee would be doing good by screening patients according to this point of view. I pointed out, however, that such a committee could act to interfere with a patient's right to agree or disagree to be human subjects in research protocols. Based on this problem, I suggested an alternative solution that I believe used both ethical principles and the ethics of caring.

This is but one example where the proposed action is driven by the well-established nursing ideal of caring. We have other examples in which caring, both in the narrower sense of giving care and in the wider sense of caring about, can be harmful. While I care and have good intentions, this caring, coupled with my good intentions, does not necessarily mean that what is best for the individual is the end result.

I would take another stand, different from that taken by Noddings. While I would want health care professionals to give me care using a caring attitude and the caring ethic, I would also want them to engage in principled thinking as well. In the real world of nursing care, as in all other worlds except in the abstract, I am suspicious of dichotomy, whether it be that of the mind-body one or of the ethics of caring versus the ethics of principles.

But to focus on the point that in order to care about and to give care, we need both of these ethics, misses another important point. As most people in the nation must know, health care is big business. To discuss whether we should support an ethics of caring or an ethics of principles overlooks the fact that often we have neither. Rather, the driving force can often be economics and the self-interest of health care professionals, the latter force fueled by malpractice concerns.

Even within the context of influencing factors in health care, there are many instances of caring. Recently I did some clinical ethics consultation with the nurses on a bone-marrow transplant unit where the ethical dilemmas are many, profound, and deeply disturbing. What came across to me was the nurses' ability to care about these patients. Because of this outpouring of being fully present to the patients, I came away with a concern about the nurses themselves. The question that lingered was: Who cares about these caring ones? One of the results of our meeting was that the head nurse and the clinical specialist decided to continue to meet with the nursing staff to discuss the communication and ethics questions that were raised. In a sense it was the beginning of a more formal caring for each other. It seems to me that while there are limits to caring, there is also a need to extend this concept to include the caring about health professionals. Perhaps the lesson here is that caring for and caring about patients can best be accomplished in an environment of caring for the caregivers. Respect for persons, which is basic to both an ethics of caring and an ethics of principles must include all persons, not just patients. The larger test of caring and principles is how we treat each other. And while more than likely we will not always succeed, it is important to keep the ideal before us and to attempt to reach it. Gandhi is remembered as saying that almost anything you do will be insignificant, but it is very important that you do it.

# References

Aristotle. 1962. *Nicomachean ethics,* translated by M. Ostwald. Indianapolis: Bobbs-Merrill.

Beauchamp, T., and J. Childress. 1983. *Principles of biomedical ethics* 2d ed. New York: Oxford University Press.

Callahan, D. 1984. Autonomy: a moral good, not a moral obsession. *Hastings Center Report* 14 (5): 40–42.

Davis, A. J. 1981. Compassion, suffering, morality: Ethical dilemmas in caring. *Nursing Law and Ethics* 2(6): 8.

Downie, R. S., and E. Telfer. 1970. *Respect for persons.* New York: Schocken Books.

Fowler, M. 1986. Ethics without virtue. *Heart and Lung* 15(5): 528–30.

Garritson, S. H., and A.J. Davis. 1983. Least restrictive alternative: Ethical considerations. *Journal of Psychosocial Nursing* 21(12): 17–23.

Jassi, A. 1977. Anarchism, autonomy and the concept of the common good. *International Philosophical Quarterly* 17: 273–83.

McIntyre, A. 1981. *After virtue.* Notre Dame, IN: University of Notre Dame Press.

Miller, B. 1981. Autonomy and the refusal of lifesaving treatment. *Hastings Center Report* 11(4): 22–28.

Noddings, N. 1984. *Caring: A feminine approach to ethics and moral education.* Berkeley: University of California Press.

Toulmin, S. 1987. The tyranny of principles. *Hastings Center Report* 11 (6): 31–39.

# Truthtelling Revisited: Two Approaches to the Disclosure Dilemma

*Sally A. Gadow, R.N., Ph.D.*

3

Two approaches to truthtelling are paternalism and advocacy. Paternalism, based on the aim of benefitting the patient, is the view that information is to be disclosed or withheld according to the anticipated effect on the patient. Advocacy, based on the aim of enhancing patient self-determination in health matters, is the view that informed decision making requires access to all information the patient considers relevant. The two ethical positions present nursing with a choice between fundamentally different moral views, a choice that will reflect the profession's underlying philosophy of care.

The issue of truthtelling is far from being solved for nursing despite trends in patient education, respect for patients' rights, and legal consent requirements. Nurses still encounter patients whose capacity for consent is limited, who insist on waiving their rights, or who probably would be harmed more than helped by disclosure. For the reductionist, there are two ways of simplifying the problem. One is a view in which candor is strictly reserved for peers and denied to patients. The other is an equally strict view in which patients are told all of the truth in all circumstances, whether or not they can bear it, understand it, use it, or want it.

For those who embrace neither of those extremes, the question is what to do with the maze in the middle. Is there a way through the complexity that is not simpleminded? Assuming that inspirational approaches are as unsatisfactory in resolving ethical issues as in addressing scientific problems, a random, situational approach is ruled out. The question then is, How can the nurse practice in an ethically coherent manner rather than base each decision on the inspiration of the moment or on a simplistic view like "never tell" or "always tell"? In answer to this question, I will compare two ethical models, advocacy and paternalism, and propose that advocacy is preferable as a moral framework for nursing practice.

First, however, it is important to recognize that what is at issue in truthtelling is not an "absolute" truth. A common objection to consent requirements is that it makes no sense to inform patients of all of the possibilities because no one can foresee them all; since no one knows the truth in that sense (except in retrospect), there is no dilemma. In other words, it is meaningless to speak of telling "the truth, the whole truth, and nothing but the truth" to a patient because it is impossible. This objection, of course, is a smoke screen. The issue is not whether to tell what no one is able to tell, rather it involves only the information that nurses do in fact possess or to which they have access. The truth behind the smoke screen is not an inaccessible, metaphysical truth; it is clinical information and judgment (Muyskens 1982). The issue is whether and when to tell patients what *is* known or believed to be the case. Even in cases in which not knowing is itself the clinical problem, the issue does not disappear. It then becomes the problem of whether to say to the patient, "I don't know."

Granting that there is always something one can tell, even if only the admission that there is not enough information on which to form a judgment, ethical guidelines can be developed for steering between the rigidity of "never tell" (or "always tell") and the randomness of inspirational ethics. The two alternatives described below may not be mutually exclusive. Situations inevitably arise in which they conflict, however, and the nurse finally must choose between them.

## Benefit Principle: Paternalism

The benefit principle dictates that nurses maximize benefit and minimize harm to patients. There will often be difficulties in deciding what is best for a patient, and patients' own notions about what is good for them are part of that difficulty. But on this view it is the professional's responsibility to make a judgment about the patient's best interest and carry out that judgment or urge the patient to do so. Information is itself one of the therapeutic options to be administered when the patient is expected to benefit, and to be withheld when the risk of harm is too great. The logical extension of this view is paternalism, in which the patient's benefit (professionally determined) is of greater importance than patient autonomy.

Applying the benefit principle then (Beauchamp and Childress 1983), the very formulation of the issue is paternalistic: How much should the nurse disclose? The question locates the responsibility for the decision with the professional rather than the patient. This approach to truthtelling is paternalistic because the patient's consent to allow the professional to withhold information cannot be obtained; the very act of seeking consent discloses to the patient that the nurse possesses (or expects to acquire) information that may not be disclosed. An example is asking the patient's permission to administer a placebo. As soon as consent is sought (except perhaps a blanket consent referring to future possibilities), suspicion is aroused and deception becomes impossible. If deception is to remain one of the therapeutic options, seeking consent is logically precluded and the approach is necessarily paternalistic (Bok 1982).

Deception is not the only therapeutic option, but until recently it has been the treatment of choice for most patients. Traditionally, professionals have emphasized the dangers of truthtelling—the risk that patients may relapse, become depressed, or even attempt suicide upon learning their prognosis. Some may become so distressed over what they perceive as an unalterable outcome that they will refuse treatment while a cure is still possible. In light of these dangers, truth has been administered with great caution.

In contrast to therapeutic conservatism toward truth, a more recent view regards candor as clinically indicated in the majority of cases. Truth then becomes the treatment of choice. Professionals believe that the greater the degree of patient assent in the healing process, the greater the chance of therapeutic success. Furthermore, deception now is seen as more dangerous than formerly—dangerous to the psychological integrity of the patient, as well as to the patient's trust in the professional and to the healing power inherent in that trust. Moreover, since it is now widely accepted that many patients intuitively sense the seriousness of their condition despite lack of information, the difficulty of effectively deceiving a patient becomes significant. As deceptive measures become more deliberate and therefore identifiable, the risk of harm from the deception increases: a patient who has been repeatedly lied to is likely to suffer greater loss of trust upon discovering the deception than a patient who simply has not been given definite information.

It must be emphasized that when the truthtelling issue is approached using the benefit principle, that is, when the nurse asks, "How much truth will benefit the patient?," *candor is no less paternalistic than deception.* In the shift from deception to disclosure, the only thing that has changed is the empirical belief regarding the therapeutic value of truth. The underlying moral premise is the same, namely, that the decision about disclosure ought to be made by the professional, according to the same criterion of benefit versus harm that is used to decide among any treatment alternatives.

## Autonomy Principle: Advocacy

The alternative approach to truthtelling is based on the value of patient autonomy. On that model, the issue is formulated differently: How much and what type of information is required for the exercise of patient decision making? Clearly this is a question that cannot be answered by the professional alone. Neither can it be answered solely by the patient, who rarely will know, without consulting a professional, the scope of relevant information available or the various possibilities for acting on that information.

This does not mean that in order for patients to exercise autonomy, they automatically should be informed of all the data that the nurse believes ought to be taken into account. That approach—I shall call it consumerism—represents the view in which the nurse mechanically supplies information. But consumerism, with its mechanical truthtelling, overlooks the fact that in selecting information that is believed pertinent to the patient, the nurse does make an important determination without the patient's consent. Thus, the consumerist approach to information is not an alternative to paternalism but a subtle vestige of it; the issue of disclosure still is resolved unilaterally by the nurse in the belief that patients are best served by administering to them the information that the professional deems pertinent. The consumerist view, in other words, is that patients ideally ought to make their decisions in the same way that professionals do.

If it is difficult to recognize that beliefs about decision making can be as prescriptive as those about health, one has only to recognize the exacting standards of professionals regarding that which they consider inappropriate in clinical decision making, specifically, the entire realm of experience characterized as the subjective, nonrational, or emotional. Thus, nurses using a consumerist approach provide strictly objective information, avoiding reference to any personal perspectives such as their own emotions or their ethical views. The tendency to provide patients with statistical probabilities as the paradigm of "truth" reflects this norm of decision making based on impersonal, quantifiable considerations.

When the truthtelling issue is given a non-paternalistic formulation ("How much and what type of information is required for the exercise of patient autonomy?"), an important misconception is avoided, one that is implicit especially in the quantitative approach: the assumption that an objective truth exists independently of the persons involved. That truth is presumed accessible to the professional, who in turn conveys it to the patient. This concept is at the heart of objections to truthtelling on the grounds that information is incomprehensible to patients. While the professional considers it imperative that patients be truthful, the possibility is overlooked that patients define or constitute for themselves the truth about their situation in a personal formulation that at times contradicts the professional's view. When such a contradiction occurs, it is interpreted as the patient being untruthful or, more benignly, as the patient's ignorance of the "real truth," an objective entity already constituted and if possible quantified, which patients may or may not understand and accept, but which they may not attempt to redefine without appearing ignorant or dishonest.

A nonpaternalistic formulation of the issue based on the value of patient autonomy assumes a different concept of truth. That is the view of truth as the most comprehensive understanding and most personally meaningful interpretation of the situation possible, encompassing subjective as well as objective realities, idiosyncratic as well as statistical tendencies, emotional as well as intellectual responses. The opposite of a truth existing independently of the persons involved, it is a truth constituted anew by the patient and nurse together. Thus it is not accessible originally to the nurse, only then to be revealed to the patient. There are of course abstract probabilities and clinical findings that a professional reveals, but whether these then define the situation for the patient—that is, whether they constitute the truth of the situation in the patient's terms—is known neither to the nurse nor to the patient until the patient has been assisted in freely making that determination. An example of the difference between statistical data and personal truth is the attempt by patients to ascertain not whether in objective terms they are dying, but whether they will be abandoned if they are dying. Thus the issue on the autonomy model is not whether to disclose to a patient *the* truth, but how best to participate with patients in defining their situation by constituting their *personal* truth.

Here the avenue most consistent with the *advocacy model* is to enable patients to determine the selection of information they wish to consider. This can be accomplished by either direct or indirect means. Direct inquiry might proceed along one of the following lines, with the nurse asking such questions as: Would you be helped in making your decision if you had more information about the clinical findings? If you knew the expected outcomes of treatment alternatives? If you knew what the prognosis is thought to be? If you knew your family's feelings on the matter? If you knew the views of persons who have faced similar decisions? A less direct way of inviting a patient to determine the extent of information needed is the expression of the nurse's own view: "I think it is helpful if people consider all of the alternatives before deciding. Do you feel this way?" In short, advocacy is the assistance to patients in determining the selection of information they wish to have, assuming of course that any information requested will be given freely and with sensitivity.

This approach to truthtelling also assumes that information other than impersonal, objective data is discussed if a patient desires (Bok 1978). Patients may wish to consider not only their own feelings and values, but those of the person caring for them. In the attempt to remedy paternalism, as well as out of a belief that only scientific data are relevant, nurses have been educated to consider such information both irrelevant and potentially coercive. On the advocacy model, however, the decision that values and feelings are irrelevant is a determination only the patient can make. While the desire not to prejudice a patient's deliberations is consistent with the autonomy principle, a refusal to disclose one's view to a patient who asks is censorship of the information a patient is allowed to have. The assumption behind the refusal is that patient and nurse are such unequal decision makers that the patient will conform to the will of the nurse. Patients indeed may conform if they are inexperienced in making health care decisions and are given no assistance in developing their autonomy. The role of the nurse in the advocacy model, therefore, is to overcome the initial inequality by assisting patients to become self-determining rather than to conform out of habit, deference, or inexperience.

The truthtelling issue is more complex on the advocacy model than the simple version of "to tell or not to tell" suggests. Its complexity is a function of the personal as well as clinical disclosure by the nurses. The ideal of advocacy is that both persons be equally or at least commensurately involved and disclosing (Gadow 1980). In other words, to the extent that the patient is addressed as a "whole person," the nurse too must be fully present. This means that, while the patient's values will be the decisive ones ultimately, the values of the nurse also may be expressed. The fear of being coercive is misplaced in the context of advocacy, for—outside of an authoritarian relationship—there is no reason to assume that communication of the nurse's values is intrinsically coercive. On the contrary, disclosure serves at least two purposes. First it provides patients with information they may find useful in understanding the nurse's clinical judgment. For example, a nurse who personally values freedom from disability over avoidance of risk may offer the judgment that the risks associated with surgery are slight and are outweighed by the benefits of restored function. The expression of such an opinion is entirely consistent with the advocacy approach, as long as two requirements are met: (a) the judgment is acknowledged to be still only abstract with respect to a specific patient's situation, because it does not yet take into account the patient's own values concerning disability and risk, and (b) the nurse's opinion is acknowledged to be personally rather than objectively true, in that it is based on the nurse's individual values (the likelihood that these will coincide with the values of most other professionals can be misleading, as if, where there is consensus, there is truth). The point here is that even the interpretation of statistics involves values: a one percent risk of death from anesthesia may be slight to a surgeon, overwhelming to the individual who fears death more than disability. The disclosure of the nurse's personal values underlying a professional judgment helps prevent both the patient and the nurse from mistaking individual values for immutable truths.

➢ A second purpose served by the expression of the nurse's values is that these represent one view of the patient's situation (one of many possible views, but ideally one that has been reached through careful reflection) that the patient may want to take into account in his or her deliberations. Just as there is no basis for assuming that a patient will concur on discovering a nurse's values, there is likewise no reason for supposing that patients would not want to consider other views in the process of forming their own.

➢ Finally, beyond providing the patient with another view to consider, the disclosure of the nurse's values signifies to the patient the nurse's commitment to the ideal of enhancing patient self-determination through thoughtful consideration of values. It is an affirmation that the nurse's involvement is commensurate with that of the patient, namely, an involvement of the person as a whole in determining that individual's unique truth.

## References

Beauchamp, T., and J. Childress. 1983. *Principles of biomedical ethics*, 2d ed. New York: Oxford University Press.

Bok, S. 1978. *Lying: Moral choice in public and private life.* New York: Random House.

Bok, S. 1982. *Secrets: On the ethics of concealment and revelation.* New York: Pantheon Books.

Gadow, S. 1980. Existential advocacy: Philosophical foundation of nursing. In *Nursing images and ideals: Opening dialogue with the humanities,* edited by S. Spicker & S. Gadow, (79–101). New York: Springer Publishing.

Muyskens, J. 1982. *Moral problems in nursing: A Philosophical investigation.* Totowa, NJ: Rowman and Littlefield.

# Caring and Gnosis: Moral Implications for Nursing

*Kathy Pike Parker, R.N., M.N.*

4

In this paper the author takes the philosophical position that the science of caring provides nursing with a core concept that lends itself to the development of a spectrum of nursing knowledge that supports the morality and excellence of the discipline. This spectrum may be conceptualized as *gnosis*, a view of knowlege that incorporates scientific information, aesthetic interpretation, and personal-intuitive experiences. A historical overview of the gnosis concept is presented, with examples of ways in which knowledge based on caring can lead to excellence in nursing education, practice, research, and theory development. Through radical reflection of the philosophical and caring literature, gnosis and caring provide a basis for the development of a novel approach to "knowing" in nursing. This approach to knowledge leads to excellence, which is a goal of practice and an ethical and moral responsibility of the nursing profession.

We are in the midst of a revolution and are privileged in many ways to witness a shift in scientific paradigms and a change in worldview. That these changes were heralded by developments in the field of physics, the favorite child of the logical positivists, is ironic. The old worldview conceptualized the whole as the sum of its parts, stressed cause and effect, was reductionistic and particularistic, separated the observer from the observed, and saw knowledge as a way to control and predict nature. Of particular interest to this discussion is the fact that many of the famous scientists responsible for initiating this longstanding scientific tradition, such as Copernicus, Newton, and Kepler, were not only scientific knowledge-seekers, but artists, mystics, and alchemists as well. The emerging worldview proposes an expanded perspective on the term *wholeness*; recognizes the connectedness among all members of humanity and between humans and the universe; addresses the importance of context, values, and probability; and equates knowledge with understanding. Although these current insights may be new in the realm of traditional scientific thought, nursing has both implicitly and explicitly incorporated these perspectives into the thinking of the discipline since the early days of Florence Nightingale.

Although nursing has been a forerunner in terms of scientific thinking, the profession traditionally has had considerable difficulty identifying its unique areas of concern. Therefore, articulating our social and moral responsibilities has been problematic. In addition, our search for nursing knowledge has been conducted not only within social, moral, and professional uncertainty, but has also been greatly influenced, as other disciplines have, by the old worldview. However, at no other time in our professional history have the phenomena of concern, the goals, and the social and moral directions of nursing been so clearly articulated as they have been in the caring literature. Caring as a core concept for nursing has identified for the profession a purpose consistent with our traditions and independent of that of medicine. Additionally, caring as the core of nursing is consistent in many regards with the new scientific paradigm and with emerging feminist theory. Nursing has the potential to empower itself through this identification.

As nursing moves ahead with caring ideas and caring perspectives, it will also shed much of the old worldview. Qualitative research, for example, has been proposed as a more appropriate method of studying caring behaviors and its effects. Self-reflection has been proposed as one method of scientific validation. Science, previously considered to be value free, has been acknowledged as value laden. Our quest for knowledge continues—knowledge of caring, knowledge of caring behaviors, and knowledge of the effects of caring relationships. Yet the use of the term *knowledge* in association with such an existential concept as caring seems somehow inadequate. It is my contention that what we are seeking is not simply knowledge in its traditional sense, but knowledge of a higher order. Furthermore, this higher order of knowledge, or *gnosis*, is important in the moral development of nursing as a caring science and discipline in two ways. First, it leads to excellence through personal and professional wholeness, which I believe is our social and moral obligation. Second, it addresses the problem of psychic malaise, or burnout, a growing problem within the profession and one which is of moral and ethical concern when we concern caring for the caregiver.

## The Concept of Gnosis

The Greek word *gnosis* simply means "knowledge," and is a term frequently associated with religious knowledge. However, gnosis in a broader sense is as old as reflection on religion itself. Traditionally, gnosis refers to a special type of knowledge needed to achieve a direct, mystical understanding of a divine Being achieved through the observation of one's own inner processes as well as from a perception of the world without. According to gnosticism, to know oneself, and thereby to know God, means to know all that there is to know. Gnosis also means knowing that a divine spark of light has been lost or covered over in this material world. As Singer writes, "For the Gnostic, the task is to find that spark and care for it and to redeem it" (1987, 11).

Most students of religion are familiar with the Gnostics, for several religious sects flourished in the Roman Empire during the first three centuries A.D. throughout Asia Minor, Syria, Palestine, Rome, Egypt, Carthage, Spain, and Gaul (Walker, 1983, 161). Wherever its followers traveled, gnosticism left a vast legacy, the full extent of which is only now coming to light. Traces of gnosticism can be found in Judaism, Christianity, Hinduism, Buddhism, and Islam. The Gnostics first appeared as an identifiable group in history when they were attacked by Christian heresiologists in the second century (Perkins 1980, 12). This persecution was the result of certain Gnostic beliefs and practices. Some of the sects were characterized by strange rituals, usually carried on in secret, which were little understood by early Christians and therefore regarded with fear and disdain. Some sects even went so far as to celebrate sensual pleasures. In addition, several of these groups were democratic, antihierarchical, and feminist in belief (French 1985, 155), tenets which were totally foreign to orthodox Christianity. As a result, members of the sects were either suppressed or wiped out, forcing the survivors underground. Since that time, gnosticism has been a nearly forgotten faith or, rather, a heresy, which is usually only studied by modern students of religion or philosophy as a point of historical interest.

Gnosticism, however, has survived, and many of its religious beliefs remain quite different from traditional Christian thought. Gnosticism integrates the concept of a Father-Mother figure as one of the persons of the Holy Trinity. Moreover, while in Christianity feminine power is subdued, in gnosticism the feminine is equal to the masculine. And unlike Christianity, which may have a more limited conceptualization of perfection as the goal, gnosticism seeks a different kind of excellence, one actualized through the achievement of *wholeness* and an acknowledgment of all human dimensions, both negative and positive. The knowledge that results from this search is called gnosis, which may in part be derived from books, but is primarily attained through life experience and self-exploration.

In a paper entitled "The Monster and the Titan: Science, Knowledge, and Gnosis" (1980), Theodore Rosak describes his conception of gnosis not as an alternative cognitive system, but as augmentative knowledge, which is different from the knowledge traditional science provides. Rosak writes that in the very beginnings of our search for knowledge "it is a certain texture of intelligibility we first and most decisively seek, a feeling in the mind that tells us, 'Yes, here is what we are looking for. This has meaning and significance' " (312). Traditional science itself arose this way when men such as Galileo, Newton, Copernicus, and Descartes developed ideas through insights achieved intuitively. It is the guiding principle of gnosis that *only* augmentative knowledge is adequate to its object, which is a strong moral statement. According to Rosak, "As long as we, at our most open and sensitive, feel there is something left over or left out of any account we give of an object, we have fallen short of gnosis. Gnosis is our awareness that, often at a level deeper than intellect, that we have not done justice to the object" (313). In other words, we may quantify, explore, and examine, but essential qualities still elude us. Thus, the achievement of excellence remains elusive.

In his paper, Rosak beautifully describes the mind as a spectrum of possibilities. Thus, gnosis, within this context, is a spectrum of knowledge. "At one end, we have the hard, bright lights of science; here we find information. In the center we have the sensuous hues of art; here we find the aesthetic shape of the world. At the far end, we have the dark, shadowy tones of religious experience, shading off into wave length beyond all perception, here we find meaning" (316). Scientific information can be thought of as shades of color in this spectrum. Artistic interpretation and personal insights also create shades in this spectrum. But gnosis is the *whole spectrum*. Nursing, through caring, can explore and address this spectrum and, thus, enhance our ability to achieve professional excellence and wholeness.

# Caring and Gnosis

Nursing has long addressed the importance of both art and science. Its procedures and interventions are often described as the scientific components of practice, while caring methods and behaviors are considered to be the artistic elements. Thus, nursing as a discipline has been described as both an art and a science. Yet, nurses know intuitively that knowledge of a higher order is crucial in expert practice. As Rosak wrote, "Gnosis is that nagging whisper at the edge of the mind which tells us, whenever we seek completeness of understanding or pretend to premature comprehension, 'not yet . . . not quite' " (1980, 313).

In *Novice to Expert* (1984), Patricia Benner also addresses the importance that this type of knowledge plays in expert nursing. She describes the expert nurse as one "who no longer relies on an analytical principle to connect an understanding of the situation to an appropriate action. The expert nurse, with an enormous background of experience, has an intuitive grasp of the situation and zeros in on the accurate region of the problem without wasteful consideration of a large range of unfruitful possibilities" (32). This type of knowledge, however, can be difficult to describe, so Benner quotes the words of an experienced, well-respected psychiatric nurse. "When I say to a doctor, 'The patient is psychotic,' I don't always know how to legitimize that statement. But I am never wrong. Because I know psychosis from inside out. And I feel that, and I know it, and I trust it" (32). These words capture perfectly the ideas of Plato, who said of this type of knowledge "There is no writing of mine about these matters, nor will there ever be one. For this knowledge is not one that can be put into words like other sciences; but after long-continued exchange between teacher and pupil, in joint pursuit of the subject, suddenly, like flashing forth when a fire is kindled, it is born in the soil and straightway nourishes itself" (*Seventh Epistle*, quoted in Rosak 1980, 309–10).

This higher order of knowledge is also consistently described in the caring literature. Indeed, it might be said that, for nursing, *caring is gnosis*, for the caring concept connotes a willingness and desire to achieve greater understanding. In her very sensitive work on caring, Nel Noddings discusses the exploration of the knowledge of things and ideas within a caring context. She writes: "In the intellectual domain, our caring represents a quest for understanding. When we understand, we feel that this object-other has responded to us" (1984, 169). She describes an active phase of knowledge-seeking that (a) depends on a store of information, (b) is analytical and (c) conveys "I'll try this," as well as a receptive mode that is intuitive, contextual, and asks "What is happening here?" She describes letting an object act upon, seize, and direct the thoughts of the knowledge-seekers so that they, in turn, can act upon the object. Noddings describes illumination as a characteristic "Eureka!" reaction. In many respects, then, Noddings's conception of knowledge is comparable with Rosak's, who writes that gnosis "is a hospitality of the mind that allows the object of study to expand itself and become as much as it might become. . . . it invites every object to swell with personal implication, to become special, wondrous, perhaps a turning point in one's life, "a moment of truth" (1980, 312). In her book *Care: The Essence of Nursing and Health* (1984), Madeleine Leininger describes scientific caring as acts and judgments of helping others based on verified knowledge. She further describes humanistic caring as those creative, intuitive, or cognitive processes based on philosophic, phenomenologic, and objective and subjective experiential feelings that help others (46). Elsewhere, she writes; "The way to understand nursing is to identify, describe, and research those central humanistic-scientific factors that are essential to effecting positive health change . . . the science of caring combines sciences with the humanities" (1979, XII). She also writes in an essay entitled "Humanism, Health, and Cultural Values" that deep humanistic aspirations are "developed and maintained through man's relationship with other men, man's relationship to a supernatural being or beings, and man's relationship to physical, psychosocial, and cultural environments" (1974, 38). These ideas demonstrate the multidimensional aspects of caring and clearly reflect the knowledge spectrum of gnosis.

The writings of Delores Gaut also reflect the concept of gnosis: "The sources of nursing science are any portions of knowledge that enter into the heart, head, and hands of nurses, and which by entering, make the performance of the nursing function more enlightened, more human, and more truly nursing" (1984, 23). She describes the importance of science, art, philosophy, and intuition in nursing, and postulates: "Maybe everything we think is part of a cosmic network, and we are a kind of "caring consciousness" for the whole system. If the notion of a cosmic consciousness is untenable, perhaps there is a collective consciousness of human beings concerned about nursing and caring and other human beings" (1984, 24). This intriguing notion of knowledge, although very metaphysical in nature, is certainly consistent with the concept of gnosis and is also consistent with the new scientific paradigm and feminist theory, which propose universal interconnectedness.

Jean Watson also addresses the importance of integrating both the humanities and science into the development of nursing knowledge. The entire spectrum of gnosis is clearly reflected in her ten carative factors. She also describes human care as an epistemic endeavor and a search for new knowledge and insights that will govern some of the ethical, intuitive, aesthetic, scientific, and methodological conditions for developing nursing as a human science (1985, 30).

## The Ethics and Morality of Gnosis

As mentioned previously, gnosticism advocates the pursuit of excellence through wholeness. It is my position that the pursuit of this type of excellence constitutes the ethical and moral foundation of the caring concept. In contrast to traditional Christianity, which regards the imitiation of God as a high virtue, gnosticism urges the acknowledgment and integration of all aspects of the individual, both positive and negative. The achievement of gnosis, or wholeness, leads to inner harmony, which facilitates the caring process. It also helps the caring individual to be "fully present" for the one cared for.

Being fully present, in the existential sense, is a concept that transcends both space and time. It is characterized by receptiveness, engrossment, and wealth, which are perceived by the one cared for even in physical absence. When the two individuals do come together in an *actual caring occasion* (Watson 1985), actions and choices are made that enrich the lives of both. As Watson writes: "What we learn from it is self-knowledge. The self we learn about or discover is every self: it is the universal-the human self. We learn to recognize ourselves in others" (1985, 59). Thus, the caring process is not only facilitated by the achievement of gnosis, but also leads to actions, choices, and moral decisions based on a caring ethic founded on gnosis.

This caring ethic differs greatly from traditional Kantian ethics in that it mandates a holistic exploration of moral dilemmas. Kant draws a distinction between acts performed out of good will or inclinication, and those done from a sense of duty (Ross 1969). Those acts done out of caring, love, and inclination are considered morally worthless. However, those acts performed out of a sense of duty are considered highly moral. Specifically, an act is done from the sense of duty, and therefore has moral worth only in one or another of the following three cases:

1. When the direct inclination is temporarily suppressed as the love of life is suppressed when our life is a very miserable one;
2. When inclination is entirely lacking, as natural sympathy is in certain people.
3. When natural inclination, though not absent, is weaker than some other inclination.

When none of these conditions is present, Kant assumes that the act proceeds from inclination, not from a sense of duty, and therefore has no moral worth. The pertinent question to be asked within the context of this discussion is, What type of knowledge would be required by an individual in order to decide to perform an act out of a sense of duty? In any of the foregoing situations, it seems that the knowledge required would necessitate either the lack or total denial of much of the gnostic spectrum.

In contrast, a caring or feminine ethic holds that acts performed out of love and inclination are highly moral. According to Noddings (1984), women, in contrast to men, prefer to discuss moral problems in terms of concrete situations. They approach moral problems not as intellectual problems but as human problems to be lived and to be solved in living. Faced with hypothetical moral dilemmas, women often ask for more information. They want to talk to those involved, feel what they feel, see what they see, and develop a sense of the total situation. With this in mind, consider again the question: What type of knowledge is required by an individual in order to decide to perform an act out of a sense of caring? I propose that gnosis, a higher order knowledge, is required to make moral and ethical decisions in a caring paradigm. Therein lies the morality of the concept.

## Moral Implications for Nursing
We can see through the work of Leininger, Gaut, Watson, and Noddings that the gnosis concept is implicit in the caring literature. What I advocate is naming that concept and making it explicit. It is through making the implicit explicit that the concept is empowered. Has not caring been implicit in nursing for generations? Have we not always been attuned to the caring needs of human beings? Yet by

addressing the caring concept explicitly, we have identified for the profession new directions, new insights, and new possibilities. In addition, we have addressed our social and moral responsibilities. Rosak writes, "It is the guiding principle of gnosis that only augmentative knowledge is adequate to its object" (1980, 313). I propose that it is the quest for gnosis within a caring paradigm that does justice to human beings, and thus it should be addressed explicitly. If gnosis is the goal, then it follows that excellence achieved through the actualization of wholeness is also the goal, and excellence, within the context of caring, is our moral and professional responsibility.

As we consider our moral responsibilities to society, we must also consider our responsibilities to ourselves. In the area of clinical practice, psychic malaise or burnout is a frequently discussed issue. Rosak (1980) addresses this problem and gives some insights in to its nature and development. It is his position that the focus on and the search for scientific information, rather than gnosis, leads to meaninglessness—and meaninglessness is a monster of our own creation, one that comes from within. He writes: "I mean an invisible demon who works by subtle poison, not upon the flesh and bone, but upon the spirit. . . . In the modern West, we have, during the past three centuries, run a dark, downhill course from an early morning humanism to a midnight humanism; from a humanism of celebration to a humanism of resignation (1980, 306). This monster prevents the professional from experiencing the intensely satisfying feelings that can come from small discoveries, small triumphs, and personal insights. Rosak refers to these feelings as "experiences of excellence" (310), which are fleeting, but extremely nourishing and replenishing. These experiences make our work personally meaningful and can serve as a goal unto themselves. He states: "If no such experience was there, then the work was not worth doing; and if it was, then why leave it out, since it must surely be the whole meaning and value of science? Once you omit that, you have nothing left except . . . information" (311). Thus, gnosis, like caring, is an important source of personal enrichment and professional sustenance.

Consider also the possibilities for developments that could be made in the nursing discipline if gnosis, rather than knowledge in its traditional scientific sense, were the goal. If we accept the gnosis spectrum as the basis of caring, it legitimizes the study of many areas often considered illegitimate in traditional scientific thought. In the area of theoretical development, a focus on gnosis could shift the goal of nursing theory from one of prediction and control to one of understanding. In addition, theory development could take place in the areas of science and aesthetics, as well as the personal and intuitive domains. The caring needs of human beings would be considered within the gnosis spectrum, but always within the context of the whole spectrum. David Bohm (1980), a philosopher and physicist, has developed a language that better describes wholeness in this context. He uses the word *re-levate* to bring to attention the notion of lifting out a certain feature from a context for consideration, but always keeping the context in mind and never separating the feature from the whole. It is through this process of re-levation that important relationships are noted, because they are always context-bound. Thus, individual theories in nursing might re-levate certain shades of the knowledge spectrum, but these shades would always be considered within the context of the entire spectrum.

Viewing clinical practice from a gnostic perspective permits multidimensional data collection, which is the most important step in the nursing process because the assessments, diagnoses, and interventions subsequently formulated can only be as sophisticated as the information initially collected. In this framework, collection of scientific information is important. However, human responses to color, art, and music are also valuable. Additionally, the intuitive, spiritual, and transcendent feelings and experiences of both the patient and the nurse become relevant. Finally, having achieved gnosis, the caring nurse could potentially identify new classes of nursing problems and develop novel, creative, and caring interventions.

In the area of nursing education, if the concept of gnosis were explored, emphasis would be placed on achieving understanding and not solely on the retention of information. As mentioned previously, Plato addressed the importance of "long-continued exchange between teacher and pupil, in joint pursuit of the subject." More attention directed at developing mentor-student relationships could not only enhance the student's knowledge, but also increase the gnostic development of the teacher and thus add more meaning to the education experience as a process. In addition, gnosis as a product of education is important in the *daily work* of nurses. Rosak writes:

Information can be exciting to collect; it can be urgently useful: a tool for our survival. But it is not the same as the knowledge we take with us into the crises of life. Where ethical decisions, death, suffering, failure confront us, or in those moments when the awesome vastness of nature presses in upon us, making us seem frail and transient, what the mind cries out for is the meaning of things, the purpose they teach, the enduring significance they give our existence (1980, 311).

The mere desire to achieve gnosis, and not necessarily its actualization, keeps open a passage through which, as Rosak says, the mind can cross over from philosophy to ecstasy and from intellect to illumination (1980, 311):

In nursing research, gnosis validates and encourages the use of many types of methodologies. Empirical, quantitative methods are valid within this system. However, qualitative methods, such as phenomenology, are equally valid. The important point here is that gnosis, a higher order of knowledge composed of information obtained in the scientific, aesthetic, and intuitive domains, can only be achieved by the use of all these methods. Thus, implicit in the concept of gnosis, is the mandate to explore problems from as many perspectives as possible. Finally, gnosis allows for the theoretical identification of new classes of conceptual and empirical nursing problems, which researchers could identify and study.

## Summary

There are many ways of knowing and many complex relationships between these ways. However, the use of the term *knowledge* seems inadequate to describe the multiple dimensions of the wisdom obtained by a caring, expert nurse. Knowledge implies scientific knowledge, not a totality of experience. I have described gnosis as a spectrum of knowledge, which includes scientific information, aesthetic interpretation, and intuitive knowledge. I have also suggested that the presence of this higher order of knowledge is implicit in the caring literature and in fact is an important feature of the caring concept. The goal of gnosis is understanding, and its achievement can lead to meaning in our personal and professional lives. In addition, the search for gnosis can lead to excellence through the achievement of wholeness, which I believe is our social and moral responsibility. Finally, I have suggested that gnosis could enrich many aspects of the nursing discipline. Rosak writes: "When the modern Prometheus reaches for knowledge, it is not the torch of gnosis he brings back or even searches for, but the many candles of information. Yet not a million of those candles will equal the light of that torch, for these are fires of a different order" (1980, 312). I believe that the torch of gnosis brings caring to nursing.

# References

Benner, P. 1984. *From novice to expert.* Menlo Park, CA: Addison-Wesley.

Bohm, D. 1980. *Wholeness and the implicate order.* London: Ark Paperbacks.

French, M. 1985. *Beyond power: On women, men and morals.* New York: Ballantine.

Gaut, D. 1984. A philosophic orientation to caring research. In *Care: The essence of nursing and health,* edited by M. Leininger, 17–25. Thorofare, NJ: Charles B. Slack.

Leininger, M. 1974. Humanism, health and cultural values. In *Health care dimensions: Health care issues,* 37–60. Philadelphia: F. A. Davis.

Leininger, M. 1979. Foreword. In *Nursing: The philosophy and science of caring,* edited by J. Watson. Boston: Little, Brown.

Leininger, M. 1984. *Care: The essence of nursing and health.* Thorofare, NJ: Charles B. Slack.

Noddings, N. 1984. *Caring: A feminine approach to ethics and moral education.* Berkeley: University of California Press.

Perkins, P. 1980. *The gnostic dialogue.* New York: Paulist Press.

Plato. *The Seventh Epistle.*

Rosak, T. 1980. The monster and the titan: Science, knowledge and gnosis. In *Introductory readings in the philosophy of science,* edited by E. Klemke, K. Hollinger and A. Kline, 305–22. New York: Prometheus.

Ross, D. 1969. *Kant's ethical theory.* Oxford: Clarendon.

Singer, J. 1987. A necessary heresy: Jung's gnosticism and contemporary gnosis. *Gnosis* 4 (11).

Walker, B. 1983. *Gnosticism.* Wellingborough, Northampshire: Aquarian.

Watson, J. 1985. *Nursing: Human science and human care. A theory of nursing.* Norwalk, CT: Appleton-Century-Crofts.

# Culture: The Conspicuous Missing Link to Understand Ethical and Moral Dimensions of Human Care

*Madeleine Leininger, R.N., M.S.N., Ph.D., L.H.D., D.S., F.A.A.N., C.T.N.* 5

In this chapter the author takes the position that culture has been the critical and conspicuously missing dimension in the study and practice of ethical and moral dimensions of human care. Culture as the totality of learned and transmitted beliefs, values, and life experiences of particular human groups is essential to generate and establish credible ethical and moral care knowledge, and to guide nursing decisions and actions. Ethical and moral care behaviors are deeply rooted in the culture's social structure, language, and environmental contexts. Nurse ethicists are challenged to discover the epistemological base of transcultural care and ethical knowledge as an integral part of humanistic and scientific nursing. Cultural examples of Western and non-Western cultures are given to show differences between and similarities of cultural values that influence ethical care lifeways. In addition, four spheres of moral and ethical care are discussed to highlight the potential areas of cultural conflicts, decisions, and actions. The author predicts that different ethical and moral codes, standards, and principles of human care will guide nursing in the future. A cadre of transcultural nurses has been carving pathways toward the discovery of transcultural care for the past three decades, but much more work lies ahead. The theory of Culture Care Diversity and Universality, with a focus on the influence of worldview, social structure factors, and environmental contexts of care, has provided many new and in-depth insights about transcultural ethical care. The author holds that it is a moral obligation of nurses to study ethical care from a transcultural perspective because our world of nursing is a multicultural one, which requires knowledge and skill of diverse cultures in order to understand and work with people of many different cultures.

Throughout the world, the topic of ethical and moral behavior of individuals, groups, governments, and cultures is of tremendous interest today, as well as of deep concern to many citizens, scholars, and students of human behavior. Diverse judgments, decisions, and actions of world leaders are being critically examined, and some negatively sanctioned if they violate ethical and moral behavior, or human rights and justice. During the past two decades, because of questionable behavior, many government officials and other public persons in the United States have been openly called into review about their ethical and moral behaviors. Governments, too, have been called to task, witness the recent questionable actions by government officials of the People's Republic of China (June 1989), which have been viewed by many people worldwide as unethical and a violation of human rights and moral justice. There has, indeed, been considerable worldwide focus on all kinds of unethical behaviors as reported in many newspapers, television programs, books, and scholarly articles during the past decade. These ethical issues, trends, and dilemmas generally reflect a worldwide cultural movement to protect human beings and to reduce actual or potential violence, death, or related human injustice.

As world cultures continue to change and interact with one another, moral and ethical dimensions of human behavior will become even more apparent in the future, with many signs of value conflicts and differences between culture beliefs, values, and lifeways. Indeed, modern modes of technology, communication, and transportation are making people realize that they are living in a rapidly changing world with many diverse cultures. A number of cultures are struggling for their own identity, special needs, ethical values, or simply to survive in this changing world. As a consequence, ethical and moral problems are increasing, and this has necessitated the need for in-depth knowledge of diverse cultures with their ethical values, codes, norms, standards, and other culturally based covenants and for the development of ethical guidelines and practices. A worldwide base of ethical and moral knowledge could well prevent intercultural problems, imprudent actions, and inappropriate cultural imposition practices. It could also lead to ways of supporting world peace and meaningful human justice.

Since the late 1970s, there has been an increased focus in nursing and medicine on moral and ethical issues, dilemmas, and problems that nurses and physicians face in providing health care services to clients. The increased number of new technologies, drugs and treatments, diverse client values, and the rise in consumer human rights are a few of the major factors leading to many ethical and moral issues in nursing and the health field. Nurses have faced these ethical issues in the most intense and continuous way because of their intimate contact with clients in providing direct care. Several nurse ethicists have identified and written about different ethical nursing issues, and they have offered philosophical views, theories, and principles to help nurses examine ethical matters in clinical practice, research, and education. The writings of Aroskar (1987), Carper (1979), Curtin and Flaherty (1982), Davis (1981), Fowler (1986), Fry (1986, 1988), Gadow (1980), Leininger (1974, 1978, 1984), Ray (1987, 1988), Veach and Fry (1987), Watson (1985), and Watson and Ray (1988) are a few of the major noteworthy ethics publications. In addition, the scholarly work of other ethicists and moral theorists with their respective viewpoints have influenced the thinking and writings of nurses, such as those of Beauchamp and Childress (1983), Callahan (1980), Gilligan (1982), MacIntyre (1981), Noddings (1984), and Toulmin (1987). Hence a beginning ethical knowledge base has been established in nursing, but nurses need to explore further established and new ethical care perspectives, and especially knowledge of diverse cultures in the world.

A systematic and comparative investigation of ethical and moral dimensions of human care of diverse cultures worldwide is one of the most challenging areas in nursing. Transcultural ethical and moral knowledge of Western and non-Western cultures is greatly needed to help nurses function effectively with people of different cultural backgrounds (Leininger 1978, 1983, 1988b). A knowledge of comparative ethical and moral values of multicultures is essential today to help nurses make meaningful care judgments, decisions, and actions. Indeed, to provide culturally congruent care and increase the client's health or well-being, culture knowledge based on ethical and moral dimensions of care is imperative. Knowing what "ought or should be" appropriate ethical care, or what is a "right or wrong" moral decision, requires that nurses know and understand different culture care values of individuals, families, groups, and institutions. Thus the challenge for nurses to be knowledgeable about and skilled in giving culturally based care to clients in the home, clinic, hospital, or in other settings is a major one, and it will increase in the future.

It is the author's position and the major thesis of this chapter that the cultural dimensions of ethical and moral behavior are the critical and conspicuously missing link in nursing education and practice. Currently, there is very limited content about the ethical and moral dimensions of culture care taught in schools of nursing, and even less emphasis in clinical practices. Cultural factors of ethical care are conspicuously missing in most nursing curricula and in clinical decisions. There are, however, implicit global assumptions and myths, as well as nursing expectations that *all* clients have the same ethical and moral human care values and must be treated alike. Cultural care differences among clients and nursing staff or with students and faculty tend to receive limited consideration, especially in ethical judgments. That cultures have different ethical and moral beliefs to guide their behavior is slowly beginning to be recognized by nurses. As a consequence, it is virtually impossible for nurses to make appropriate decisions about individual clients, families, or groups without respect to the client's specific cultural values, beliefs, and lifeways (Leininger 1970, 1978, 1983).

This critical absence of culturally based ethical and moral care knowledge in nursing is largely related to the limited educational preparation of nurses in transcultural nursing, anthropology, the humanities, or in comparative philosophical and social science fields. Accordingly, nurses and especially nurse ethicists, tend to overlook the significant role that culture plays in ethical and moral behavior or decisions regarding human care. Some nurse ethicists deliberately avoid the concept of culture and instead assume universal ethical principles, codes, covenants, and standards of human behavior. This lack of substantive knowledge about cultural differences in ethical values among world cultures greatly limits the establishment of a systematic and epistemological foundation for ethical care.

There has also been a tendency among Western nurse ethicists to believe that our Western ethical philosophies, values, and practices exist worldwide, or that they are applicable to non-Western cultures in professional nursing practice. This ethnocentric premise fails to recognize non-Western ethical values and practices that are extremely important to non-Western peoples and especially to non-Western nurses and how they view nursing and practice in making ethical decisions. Such marked ethnocentric views lead to cultural imposition practices, which have serious ethical and moral implications (Leininger 1978). Hence, one of the most critical, longstanding, and conspicuously missing links in nursing has been the lack of knowledge and study of the cultural dimensions of ethical and moral care. And as our society becomes increasingly multicultural, clients will expect that their ethical values and moral beliefs will be respected and acted upon appropriately by health personnel. This means that nurses must become knowledgeable about different cultures, discover ethical aspects of human care, and be aware of how different cultures reach ethical and moral decisions.

The purpose of this chapter is to discuss the importance and significance of culture. It is the critical basis for knowing, understanding, and generating a body of ethical and moral knowledge of human care. This knowledge can be used to make ethical decisions in human care practices. I take the position that transcultural ethical and moral care knowledge is imperative to establish any credible, accurate, and meaningful way to help clients of diverse cultures. For without ethical culture care knowledge, nurse clinicians, theoreticians, researchers, and educators would be "functioning in the dark," unable to make meaningful and reliable ethical and moral decisions about human care or to establish accurate ethical care knowledge. Moreover, establishing substantive knowledge of ethical cultural differences and similarities between Western and non-Western cultures is essential to advance worldwide nursing knowledge and practices.

There is no concept so powerful and so meaningful to clients in the caring, healing, or dying process as knowing and sensitively using their culturally based ethical and moral values. Nurses, and especially nurse ethicists, must take active and deliberate steps to study ethical values, beliefs and practices of worldwide cultures, so that this body of knowledge can be used in nursing education and practice. The author holds that her theory of Culture Care Diversity and Universality, and the use of qualitative research methods continue to be one of the most helpful means to discover and understand the meanings of ethical and moral culture care (Leininger 1978, 1985b, 1988a). Accordingly, this chapter deals with the author's position of the importance of nurses' discovering and understanding the ethical and moral dimensions of human care. Several transcultural nursing and anthropological examples of cultural care differences are presented to show cultural variabilities of ethical-moral human care.

## Rationale for and Importance of Culture to Discover the Epistemics of Ethical and Moral Care

The rationale for establishing culturally based ethical and moral knowledge about human care is to ensure that nurses will understand and be able to make appropriate decisions in the care of individuals, families, and groups from different cultural backgrounds, for if the nurse's ethical care judgments are not reasonably congruent with the clients', a host of unfavorable problems can occur. From the growing body of transcultural nursing knowledge of diverse cultures, one finds that some clients avoid nurses and other health personnel who do not understand or value their ethical cultural beliefs and lifeways (Horn 1978; Leininger 1970, 1978, 1984, 1988a). Some clients do not cooperate or comply with professional decisions that are against their ethical or moral values. Still other clients may comply under duress during an emergency, but their well-being, recovery, or healing may be affected. There are other clients who may press legal suits when their cultural values are not respected or honored.

Most assuredly, the evolving discipline of nursing needs an epistemic ethical and moral knowledge base that takes into account cultural differences and similarities in order to provide knowledgeable and accurate judgments that are congruent with clients' values and lifeways (Leininger 1988a). No longer should nurses assume that ethical or moral codes, covenants, principles, standards, or rules of behavior are universal. Presently there are indications that more cultural variability is evident worldwide than are universal features of ethical codes and norms of human behavior. This trend toward cultural diversity is likely to increase in the next century as today's minority cultures become tomorrow's dominant cultures and as other cultures assert their special identities and values. Even today most cultures generally strive to preserve many of their traditional values while selectively choosing new ones. Nurses need to be knowledgeable about both traditional and changing cultural values and sensitive to the fact that some cultures might fight valiantly to preserve or change specific values for a variety of reasons.

In the epistemic pursuit of transcultural care knowledge, nurse ethicists should consider these questions: (1) What is universal about ethical care or the ethics of nursing? (2) What are the diverse beliefs, meanings, forms, expressions, symbols, metaphors, and other manifestations of ethical and moral care?; (3) What could explain the differences in cultural patterns and themes of ethical care?; (4) How do particular cultures interpret or explain their values of ethical care decisions?; (5) In what ways do the language, the environment, and social structure factors influence ethical care practices?; (6) What existing care knowledge can be tapped from the transcultural nursing research of diverse cultures from the past three decades?; (7) How does the culture in the home, hospital or clinic, or institution influence the clients' and nurses' ethical decisions?; and (8) How useful is medical ethics for developing nursing ethics or the ethics of care? These questions and others make one realize that nursing is at the frontier of discovering ethical care knowledge from a transcultural perspective. It also makes one realize our limited knowledge of transcultural ethical care and question the usefulness of biomedical knowledge in nursing, as nurses focus on human care as the essence and central domain of nursing (Leininger 1983, 1984, 1988c; Watson 1985).

Theoretical knowledge or ideas about care may come from several different disciplines to develop ethical nursing care knowledge, but one potentially rich source is anthropology. Anthropologists have been studying cultures for more than a hundred years, and they have discovered that culture is a powerful construct to explain human values and behaviors. The early work of Boas (1966), Herskovits (1964), and Kluckhohn (1970), and the more recent work of Downing and Kushner (1988), Haviland (1987), Lanham (1986), and other anthropologists support this statement. Anthropologists have been intrigued to discover how different cultures have created and maintained certain ethical and moral rules, rights, and sanctions over time to maintain justice and peace, or to survive. Anthropologists have also discovered that cultures vary greatly in ethical rules and expressions of human justice and rights (Downing and Kushner 1988).

Transcultural nurse researchers have also been studying the way cultural values, beliefs, and practices influence ethical care and health behavior since the early 1960s (Leininger 1970, 1978, 1984, 1988b; Luna 1989; Horn 1978; and Wenger 1988). For example, in Luna's research (1989), she found that Arab-Lebanese Muslim women viewed it as unethical for Anglo-American nurses to press for "bonding" between a newborn infant and the father in hospital nursing care practices. Wenger (1988) found that among Old Order Amish it was considered unethical practice for a child to be separated from his or her mother or a maternal kinswoman while the child was hospitalized. Leininger (1978) discovered that the Gadsup people in the Eastern Highlands of New Guinea would consider a nurse unethical if the nurse revealed sex secrets that belonged only to women. These and other examples can be found in the transcultural nursing literature.

Transculturally prepared nurses and anthropologists have been aware of such moral and ethical cultural differences and have frequently taken stances or shared this information with outsiders in order to protect or clarify the expressions of ethical acts related to violence, feuds, infanticides, circumcisions, and other behaviors of specific cultures. Ethical values about abortions and infanticide vary considerably in different cultures. In the early 1960s, I well remember that the Gadsup villagers of the Eastern Highlands of New Guinea were stunned to hear that Western women had abortions, as the Gadsup greatly valued life and actively protected newborns. Moreover, they did everything possible to have a viable and healthy infant and to see it remain healthy. Or consider the Eskimos who do not consider a fetus as human until named, and so practiced infanticide until recently. The ethical view of the Eskimos would contrast with "pro-life" supporters in the U.S. who do not consider abortion morally permissible because the fetus is human from the time of conception. Such major cultural differences obviously have moral and ethical consequences that nurses need to know and understand in order to care for clients of different cultures.

As nurses study different cultures, they are challenged to search for both universal and diverse dimensions of moral or ethical aspects of human care. My theory of Culture Care Diversity and Universality provides a broad framework within which to search for differences and similarities with the worldview, social structure, and environmental factors that tend to influence cultural care variations (Leininger 1985a, 1988a). As nurse researchers use the theory, they search for evidence and explanations of transcultural variations in ethical and moral behavior, looking for culture-specific and universal features. They especially seek *emic* (local) data from cultural informants in order to get accurate interpretations or explanations of culture-specific values and behaviors, and reflect on these feelings with *etic* data that comes from outsiders' views and professional values. Getting to the *emic* (or insider's) worldview and ethical posture is essential to prevent inaccurate interpretations by outsiders (the *etic* view). It usually helps the nurse see and compare two different sets of data or viewpoints, and helps to prevent or reduce cultural imposition nursing practices (Leininger 1985a, 1985b).

Another closely related challenge for nurse researchers in discovering transcultural ethical care phenomena is to examine Western and non-Western comparative philosophies and classification systems of ethical care. Nurses may not realize that our Western normative (or non-normative), descriptive, utilitarian, deontological, and other classificatory typologies may not exist in non-Western cultures. In fact, most nurse ethicists in the U.S. assume that these are universal ethical principles and typologies, but there is still limited evidence that this exists transculturally. From my three decades of transcultural field research, I have found that many non-Western cultures classify, know, and interpret ethical care behavior quite differently from our Western society due to differences in worldview, social structure, and other cultural factors (Leininger 1983–1989). Western nurses can make inaccurate and inappropriate judgments about non-Western behaviors if they do not know non-Western ethical types and how the cultures know and interpret their *emic* types. One also wonders how nurses can teach and promote universal ethical care principles and codes without knowing such worldwide cultural differences. Knowledge about how each culture knows and classifies ethical and moral care is essential to develop the epistemics of ethical and moral care knowledge. It is, therefore, difficult for nurse ethicists to write about ethical care without knowledge of cultural universals and variabilities, and how cultures explain their ethical and moral decisions or actions. Currently, very little has been documented by nurses about Western and non-Western ethical and moral views of human care and their influence on health, well-being, illness, disability, or death.

Another related and major concern in nursing is the problem of *cultural imposition.* I have defined cultural imposition as the tendency of nurses to impose their values, beliefs, and practices on another culture (Leininger 1978, 490). This practice often occurs due to the nurses' lack of awareness about different cultures and nurses' ethnocentric tendencies. Cultural imposition usually leads to client dissatisfaction, non-compliance, stresses, and a host of other ethical problems that limit the client's well-being. Ethnocentrism, believing that one's own values are the best, most desired, or preferred, is at the root of cultural imposition (Leininger 1970, 1978). Today there are a host of cultural imposition problems that need to be identified and handled for therapeutic and ethical outcomes in nurse-client care. Unfortunately, cultural imposition practices are not always recognized unless nurses have transcultural nursing knowledge and respect clients' culture background and needs. When the negative consequences of cultural imposition are recognized, nurses will find that clients are extremely relieved, and their recovery process is often accelerated. Nursing is not alone in cultural imposition practices; other health disciplines suffer from the same lack of awareness.

To advance ethical care knowledge and to reduce the serious and growing problems related to cultural imposition, the nurse should consider these questions: (1) What are the ethical consequences of cultural imposition practices on the health and well-being of clients and their families?; (2) How can nurses with ethnocentric values, biases, and prejudices prevent cultural imposition practices?; (3) Under what clinical contexts do cultural imposition practices tend to occur, and why?; (4) How can nurses become aware of their cultural imposition practices?; and (5) What are schools of nursing doing to prevent non-therapeutic ethnocentrism and cultural value imposition practices with students? In general, answers to these questions could help reduce or prevent unfavorable ethnocentric and cultural care imposition practices in nursing.

Today many nurses work in foreign cultures with cultural strangers and in unfamiliar communities. The need for transcultural nursing knowledge and skills is clearly evident in such situations. Learning about cultural sanctions and taboos of different cultures can help nurses discover ethical care values and guidelines for care practices. Transcultural nursing and anthropology courses have been essential to help nurses discover ethical care knowledge, reduce ethnocentrism, and to provide culturally congruent ethical care decisions. In fact, nurses who have been prepared in transcultural nursing have been most grateful to know about cultures before they begin to work with them as it has prevented a host of culture problems (Leininger 1983, 1989). Most importantly, such preparation has prevented cultural imposition practices and reduced cultural stresses and conflicts in the care of cultural strangers. In the future all nurses must be prepared in basic and advanced transcultural nursing courses and degree programs, because clients will be more active and demand that their culture values and ethical rights be respected. Transcultural ethical insights will also prevent many legal problems and nurse-client conflicts.

In considering further the importance of culture to discover the epistemics of ethical caring and non-caring behavior, I have found from my research that care behaviors tend to be covert and often buttressed in the worldview, social structure, cultural context, and in the non-verbal expressions of cultural behaviors (Leininger 1970, 1983, 1984, 1988b). Epistemologically, the sources of ethical and moral care tend to be embedded especially in the worldview, religion, kinship, economic, and technological aspects of behavior, but with variabilities in Western and non-Western cultures. Ethical and moral care concepts have to be teased out of informant's worldviews, philosophical ideas, and recurrent behaviors with their meanings and uses. In addition, cultural symbols, metaphors, expressive, behaviors, and specific contexts are valuable sources to confirm accurately caring and non-caring ethical and moral behaviors. Discovering the covert or hidden ethical care behaviors requires not only considerable knowledge about a culture, but also ethnonursing interviewing skills and much patience in order to let informants provide *their* explanations or interpretations of what constitutes ethical or non-ethical care behaviors. The researcher must be extremely careful not to make premature ethical judgments or interpretations based on the researcher's biases, *etic* professional perspectives, and values. Cultural informants are often hesitant to share their ethical values because of the fear that health professionals might misinterpret, demean, or think less of them.

Comparative insights of ethical care differences and similarities among clients often provide clues to cultural changes and new theoretical ideas to advance a science of ethical care. For example, ways to provide comfort care in relieving pain vary with Anglo-Europeans compared with Vietnamese clients. Comparative ethical knowledge means understanding that individual client's care ideas, but also seeking patterns and themes of ethical values and care behaviors of families, communities, corporations, and public and private cultural institutions. Comparative ethical care knowledge means focusing on a number of different cultures to discover commonalities and differences for a science of ethical human care. Discovering and contrasting the differences between and similarities among specific care constructs such as touch, succorance, enabling, comfort, nurturance, and helping with Western and non-Western cultures, is already providing one of the richest epistemic knowledge sources about human care in nursing and about an ethics of care (Leininger 1984, 1988b). The continued search for diverse and universal patterns of ethical care requires a rigorous comparative ethnomethods approach in order to study care in all cultures worldwide and over time. It requires the use of precise linguistic terms and cultural documentation of *emic* interpretations of care phenomena to account for variabilities or diversities. But once this goal is achieved, nursing will have a substantive and reliable body of ethical care knowledge, which can be used to teach comparative ethical care. It will help future nurses and clinicians make care decisions that support *culturally congruent care*—care that fits the client's beliefs, practices, and well-being (Leininger 1988a).

Most importantly, this transcultural body of care knowledge can be used to establish a meaningful and credible basis for ethical care principles, standards, codes, and guidelines for the nursing profession. Outdated and inaccurate ethical codes and standards of today can then be replaced with culture specific and universal guides of ethical care knowledge. Universal and non-universal ethical care principles will be used by nurses to accommodate clients who have different cultural values and to reduce non-compliant client behaviors. Nurses will also be able to use this knowledge to adapt to ethical care changes of cultures and of different health care institutions whose ethical values change over time. While nurses may find very few ethical care universals, they will have care diversities to guide their practices. However, they must be alert to the fact that some traditional cultures will want to preserve their own distinct ethical and moral principles as it gives them more stability, cultural identity, and security. While other cultures may find new values "intriguing", they can also easily relinquish them, especially technological ethical values. Nursing is far from achieving a body of transcultural ethical care universal or non-universal knowledge, but major efforts must continue to be directed toward that goal, and transcultural nurses and ethical care theorists can lead the way.

## Some Culture Specific Ethical and Moral Care Values

It is always fascinating for nurses to realize that most cultures in the world explicitly or implicitly teach sets of cultural values to guide people in their moral commitments and to uphold desired ethical behavior. Diverse enculturation processes and sanctions exist to ensure proper moral and ethical culture behavior. Some cultures are quite conscientious in teaching and monitoring ethical behavior throughout the life cycle; other cultures, such as the United States, tend to be less conscientious in their enculturation practices. In Japan, the subject of ethics and morality has been taught for a longer period of time than in the United States. In a course called *Dotoku* (referring to ethics), students receive ethical and moral instruction related to group perseverance, diligence, quietness, patience, respect for elders, and teamwork (Lanham 1986). These values are mainly derived from their social structure and worldview, but especially from their religious and kinship systems. Japanese ethical values have guided the people in decision making and actions for many years, with only slight changes. The Japanese culture shows tenacity in the teaching of ethical values and principles, which has promoted cultural identity and other benefits to their sociocultural institutions.

In the United States, I have studied Japanese-American individual and family behavior in different nursing contexts, and have identified some behaviors similar to those mentioned above, such as the ethical care value of deference to and respect for the elderly, reciprocal kindness to one another, benevolence, and a tendency to forgive easily (Leininger 1983–1989). The dominant ethical care value of Japanese families to show *respect for the elderly* was clearly apparent in the home and in hospitals. In fact, deference and respectful care were viewed as a moral responsibility for nurses as caregivers with first, second, and third generation Japanese elderly and middlescent informants. While some slight variations prevailed with these ethical care values, they remained dominant themes of Japanese-American belief and action.

In an industrial context, the ethical values of *respect* and *deference* were identified as important in a large Japanese manufacturing plant in the Midwest, where many employees had recently come directly from Hiroshima, Japan. They spoke English and Japanese, and were extremely deferent and benevolent to all Japanese employees, especially older employees in authority positions. They showed strong reciprocal loyalty and respect for one another and a "family-like corporate loyalty." These values were predominant ethical care values in the management of the Japanese plant. The Japanese company president was much respected for his role with employees who were deferent to him in many ways. The president's ethical caring behaviors of mutual respect for all employees was readily identified. This care value greatly attributed to group employee solidarity and a desire among employees to achieve the stated institutional goals rather than individual employee achievements or awards. The few Anglo-American employees in the plant had difficulty at first adjusting to the Japanese ethical care values because their values of *high individualism, competition, self-reliance,* and *less respect for those in authority* were in conflict with the Japanese care values. These two markedly different sets of ethical care values had been a covert source of tension and conflict as the Anglo-American employees were the minority employees. With consultation through group discussion, the employees became aware of these transcultural value difference and began to deal successfully with ethical care differences. The dominant action plan of *care accommodation,* as reflected in my theory goals, proved to be helpful in decreasing intercultural tensions between the two groups (Leininger 1988a).

Another illustration of the meanings and expressions of ethical care was discovered in Luna's recent study (1989) of Arab-Lebanese Muslims in three urban culture contexts. This was a major longitudinal study covering a three-year period, which I monitored as a research consultant and mentor. The purpose of the study was to identify the meanings and expressions of culture care, including moral and ethical care behaviors. It soon became apparent that all ethical and moral decisions were clearly derived from the Qur'an. The Qur'an is the holy scripture that contains the tenets of the Islamic religious beliefs and practices, and it guides Arab-Muslim beliefs care and practices. Luna found that care was viewed as *responsibility* and a *universal moral obligation* with all informants. There were, however, some gender role differences. The ethical care expectations for the male Arab-Lebanese Muslims were *honor, protection,* and to be an *economic provider* and *protector* of the Lebanese family. In contrast, the female Lebanese-Arab Muslims emphasized and practiced care as *family honor, unity,* and a *social and domestic family responsibility.* These ethical care responsibilities were clearly embedded in the religious and kinship systems. They were taught at an early age to children and served as a moral care guide to their daily living. These ethical care values became of central importance in helping nurses give culturally congruent care to Arab-Lebanese Muslims.

Prior to the research, hospital and clinic nurses and physicians were unaware of these *culture-based ethical care values* and had been frustrated in trying to get clients to cooperate, comply, or to understand what the staff wanted them to doo. Cultural imposition and ethnocentric practices were identified, as were client dissatisfactions. Avoiding professional-staff appointments had been a common practice of Arab clients because it was perceived that the staff offered inappropriate and questionable care practices. There were other specific ethical care expectations of the Arab clients that made them uncomfortable with physicians and nurses. These were closely related to their religious beliefs and cultural values, such as the nurse giving medications to them with her left hand and a lack of attention to the modesty of the females. The nursing and medical staff in the hospital and clinic context needed culture-specific care knowledge in order to provide meaningful care to Arab-Lebanese Muslims, and thus protect their cultural values and rights. Luna's transcultural research findings are now being used by nurses in the care of Arab-Lebanese clients and families, and clients are responding positively.

Both Luna's (1989) and Wenger's (1988) research studies are examples of in-depth ethnonursing research in discovering similarities and differences in ethical care values and of the need for culture specific care practices. These transcultural findings are helping to build knowledge to support *ethical specific care decisions and actions.* The research methods of ethnonursing and ethnography and the Cultural Care theory were extremely important and valuable to discover and confirm ethical care meanings and patterns of behavior of different cultures (Leininger 1985a, 1988a).

In the search to identify universals or commonly shared care knowledge, a few examples will be offered from my research (1983–1989) with Mexican-Americans, North American Indians, Chinese-Americans, Arab immigrants, and Vietnamese refugees. These cultures all shared the common ethical care values of *filial respect and obedience* especially to the elderly. There were some slight differences in patterns of their care expression and in the meanings from their experiences that guided their ethical cultural care behaviors. For example, the Chinese-American informants had been in America for five years, and they retained a strong ethical obligation to be *obedient* and *compliant* to government officials and to the elderly. This finding, however, was not as strongly evident in the other four cultures. But ethical care variability was clearly evident with the values of *filial respect for* and *obedience to the elderly* with all five cultures and between first and second generations. In each of the five cultures, there were explicit prescriptions for what "ought to be" or "should be" desired ethical caring behavior and moral commitments of what made their actions "right" or "wrong" (Leininger 1983–1989). The informants were able to identify and explain the meanings of ethical care expectations, but it required that the researcher sensitively tease out the embedded care values from their religious, kinship, and lived-through cultural values. Currently, these ethical care values are being used to provide culture specific nursing care to individuals and families of these five cultures.

In the hospital context, it was interesting to discover that Anglo-American nurses showed less evidence of overt respect for clients of the five cultures cited above and for Anglo-American elderly. For many Anglo-American hospital nurses, care of the elderly was viewed as a "duty" or "task," and they expressed a preference to care for young or middle-aged clients. Several nurse informants were encouraging the elderly to be *self-reliant* and to be *self-care givers* as they had been taught Orem's self-care theory. Interestingly, the nursing ethic of self-care was very difficult for these elderly clients to accept, as it as incongruent with their cultural values and ethical expectations (Leininger 1983–1989). The Anglo-American nurses were curious about the Vietnamese and Chinese clients and tended to avoid them because they could not speak their language and did not know their culture. Because of the nurses' lack of cultural knowledge and language uses, they were greatly handicapped in giving appropriate culture care to clients of the five cultures.

In general, discovering and using appropriate ethical and moral culture care knowledge can make a major difference in ways nurses can help clients to restore their health and well-being. Knowledge of culture specifics and universals about ethical and moral care behaviors remains largely undiscovered. Research findings from diverse cultures world wide should help open the door to new modes of nursing care decisions and actions. This discovery is just beginning and will take time and diligent efforts with over two thousand cultures in the world.

Interestingly, the ethical concepts of autonomy, self-respect, and human dignity are frequently cited as universals in the nursing literature and in the Code of Ethics for Nursing (Viens 1989), however, the existence, meanings, and expressions have not been *established* by research as cultural universals. While the nursing profession undoubtedly would like to have ethical values serve as "universal" guides to nurses' behavior and actions, the epistemic cultural knowledge base with its cultural variabilities has not been verified. It is, therefore, important that nurses begin to study Western and non-Western cultures to establish the substantive foundation for ethical care constructs, meanings, and expressions. This is one of several transcultural nursing goals which the author and her graduate students have been working toward using the Theory of Culture Care with its many practical and abstract features to provide culturally congruent care.

Most importantly, ethical care concepts, principles, and practices need to be taught in schools of nursing so that nurses can learn and skillfully use ethical care concepts with clients, families, and groups of different cultural backgrounds. To achieve this goal, some major changes in nursing curricula are needed to replace vague, ethnocentric, or inaccurate ethical concepts that do not reflect diverse or similar culture values. Teaching *emically-derived* culture care knowledge is essential for beneficial client outcomes and to deal with the nurse's *etic* views derived from the profession, which may not always fit with the client's care values. Transcultural nurse specialists and generalists can be of a great help in establishing relevant teaching content and curricular changes (Leininger 1989). The use of the growing body of transcultural nursing care findings could help to advance the science of ethical care. In addition, Culture Care Theory and ethnonursing research methods are invaluable to advance the explication of specific ethical moral dimensions of care that are rooted in culture values and lifeways. As clients continue to seek culture-congruent care to support their ethical and moral care beliefs, one can anticipate that all professional nurses will need transcultural care knowledge in their teaching, curricular work, and clinical practices. In general, a major gap exists in regard to ethical and moral care largely because there are still too few faculty and nurse researchers prepared in transcultural nursing, and who value ethical cultural variabities in nursing.

## Contextual Spheres of Ethical Culture Care

In this final section, four contextual spheres of ethical and moral culture care will be briefly discussed from different perspectives: (a) *personal or individual,* (b) *professional or group,* (c) *institutional or community,* and (d) *cultural or societal.* These four spheres can be viewed as differential contexts, which give meaning to and greatly influence ethical and moral decisions and actions of care. They are the reality contexts or perspectives in which nurses and clients function, and which need to be recognized in order to understand and accurately assess ethical care. These four contextual spheres of knowing and understanding can guide the nurses' thinking and actions in ethical and moral decisions. They can also increase nurses' competencies and effectiveness as they realize that differential contexts can mean shifts in the way nurses function in caring for clients, families, or groups of people.

In considering these contextual spheres of ethical and moral behavior, nurses need to recognize the principle that different contexts can lead to different meanings and behaviors (Leininger 1970, 1978, 1984, 1988b). Each sphere reflects different cultural frames of reference for ethical care decisions and actions. For example, in the United States, Americans maintain a dominant focus on the *individual* or *one's personal views, rights, beliefs, and actions,* and ethical decisions tend to be referenced to *individuals* as the sphere of knowing or understanding. In contrast, in the People's Republic of China, the Chinese maintain a dominant reference to *collective* and *societal norms* in any decision or action, and personal or individual rights receive limited attention and are not of prime consideration. Indeed, individual rights in China are deferred to what is "best for society," or the *collective societal good.* Any decisions regarding individual rights become part of a communal obligation and a right of the central government, based on well-known and explicit cultural rules and regulations (Leininger 1983–1989). Thus any individual ethical rights and freedoms in China are of limited importance and deferred to the collective needs in the Chinese society with reinforced rules, sanctions, and obligations.

These care expectations were identified in the author's research with the dominant Chinese culture care values of *obedience* and *compliance* within the country and for recent Chinese living in the United States. Interestingly, these cultural values were evident during the recent (June 1989) pro-democratic students' movement in China in which the central political committee of the communist government (Politburo) denied any individual or personal wishes of students as they rallied for a more democratic government. Such strong collective central government rules were alarming to many Americans and especially to American students who greatly value freedom and the rights of individuals to be heard, to make choices, and to receive due consideration of their needs. For American students, the Chinese cultural norms or rules of *obedience, compliance,* and *deference to authority* were extremely difficult to accept; however, the Chinese students in the People's Republic of China should have been keenly aware of them. It was interesting to find in my study that Chinese-American students, who had come from China since 1980 and who were studying at a Midwestern university, had retained these values of obedience to the government as an obligation, but they were also looking for future changes toward more democratic principles when they returned to China (Leininger 1983–1989).

Turning to the Western world of nursing, especially in the United States, the nurse's individual and professional values and perceived personal rights are dominant spheres that tend to govern what nurses should or ought to be. In the culture of Western nursing, most nurses become upset and protest today if their perceived individual or professional rights are violated (Leininger 1970, 1984). Collectivities, institutions, or group values are often viewed with suspicion, especially if individual rights are perceived to be threatened. Many ethical issues, conflicts, and dilemmas become major problems to the nurse when his or her individual rights and autonomy are not fully considered. The nurse usually has to deal with at least three major sets of ethical rights. First, there are the *personal* home culture values that the nurse learned when growing up in the family culture. Second, there is the *professional set of cultural values* that the nurse learns in schools of nursing. Third, the nurse is expected to live by and value the *American or societal cultural values* as a U.S. citizen. The latter contextual sphere is important for the nursing profession to become culturally and socially relevant to humanity. In addition, the nurse is also challenged by the *public or private institutional value system* of hospitals, agencies, or wherever the nurse is employed. These different sets of cultural and ethical values often differ greatly, and nurses can experience cultural value conflicts or stresses. Cultural conflict in ethical values is often a major reason for nurse turnover or resignation, but it is not always recognized. Hence the nurse can get caught in different contextual ethical spheres of knowing and experiencing what is "good" or "bad," or "right" or "wrong", or what threatens the nurses autonomy or rights. These different cultural contexts of ethical knowing need to be recognized by nurses to prevent cultural burnouts, cultural imposition practices, cultural conflicts, and even serious legal problems.

In these different contextual spheres of ethical thinking and decision making, the nurse may need to *compromise* personal ethical values for another perceived good or benefit. Sometimes the nurse works out what Ray (1988) calls a "bonding" relationship with the client. Sometimes, the nurse avoids ethical dilemmas by not dealing with them or figuratively "running away from" the ethical conflicts. And sometimes nurses live almost perpetually with unresolved ethical care conflicts that reduce their energies, freedoms, professional skills, and work satisfaction.

Turning to clients, I found from my research that their ethical and cultural values were limitedly assessed by nurses, but the clients were fairly quick to identify by "trial and error" the institutional rights, standards, or rules of hospital behavior (Leninger 1983–1989). The clients' personal and cultural care beliefs and values tended to get limited attention by the hospital staff. If clients acquiesced to nurses, physicians, or institutional ethical norms, they showed some signs of being restless and dissatisfied if the norms were counter to their values. It was also difficult for the nurse and physician to fully accept and respect clients' right to choose. In the hospital context, clients often had to yield to professional staff's values and choices or to the institution norms because of fear that they would not receive any care or treatment if they asserted their own rights or choices. The client, therefore, tended to comply with health personnel's desires to get reasonable care and treatment. This is a critical ethical issue today with the extreme shortage of nurses, with many acutely ill clients in the hospital, and with short-term hospital stays, as clients may often feel that they are "at the mercy of nurses and physicians." Clients know they are not on their "home turf," able to make safe decisions or to assert their rights. Several clients told me that it was "almost impossible to refuse whatever was offered by the nurse or physician because if they did not comply they would not be able to remain in the hospital for treatment or care. Or, if they did not comply they would be treated in a non-caring way" (Leininger 1983–89). Thus the client's decision was usually to comply. Those ethical issues and other related ones merit further study and resolution by nurses and physicians.

It has also been interesting to note that in some cultures, such as the Philippine, Korean, and mainland Chinese, clients want and expect the physician and nurse to make decisions for them, especially when they are critically ill, because of their cultural value of *deference* to those in authority. However, most American clients take a different position and want to make choices and decisions as *their* ethical American right and freedom. Today many American clients are becoming more active in choosing their hospitals, therapists, treatments, and care. The "Patient's Bill of Rights" is a document often given to clients as they enter the hospital, but ethical conflicts prevail between the nurse and client when their different ethical rights cannot be successfully resolved or compromised. In contrast, non-American clients are often baffled by the Anglo-Americans assertive demands for their rights and freedoms in client services. In the future, these major cultural differences in values and in ethical and moral viewpoints need to be considered in order to provide quality nursing care.

Given these differential contextual spheres that influence the nurse's ethical decisions, how does and should the nurse resolve them? What are appropriate or inappropriate ethical decisions in these different contextual spheres and with different client and nurse expectations? Is there a hierarchical ordering in which one sphere supersedes the other in different cultures? Do cultural or societal values have rights over personal, individual, or institutional rights in different cultures? What happens if the "traveling nurse" follows the Western type of utilitarian ethics in a non-Western culture? How will this nurse know what is "good for the utility," or for the assumed majority of clients in the particular cultures in which employed? Or, if the nurse makes an ethical care decision from the *deontological* stance, how congruent is this decision for what is "best for the individual" unless the nurse knows the individual's cultural values, beliefs, and practices, let alone the societal cultural values? Do current public health policies violate culture values? These are additional untapped ethical nursing questtions that merit systematic study as important ethical and moral care issues related to ethical care.

As nurses become knowledgeable about Western and non-Western cultural philosophies, they will be able to develop comparative and new ethical theories, principles, codes, covenants, and practices. But until this body of knowledge becomes explicated, it will be difficult to provide culturally based ethical care. Most assuredly, nursing researchers using qualitative research methods such as phenomenology, ethnonursing, ethnography, grounded theory, symbolic interaction, and other methods within the qualitative paradigm will be essential because ethical and moral care values are almost impossible to measure, manipulate, experimentally control, or arrive at through the linear or positivistic logical reasoning that characterizes the quantitative paradigm (Leininger 1985b). Both subjective and objective ethical care concepts, principles, and patterns need to be sought, from the *people's* worldview, philosophical ideologies, and cultural values.

In this chapter, I took the stance that culture is the conspicuous and critically missing link to discover and understand the ethics of care and nursing, and that ethical and moral meanings and expressions are epistemologically rooted in culture. Culture, I contend, provides the broadest holistic knowledge base to build an accurate and reliable knowledge base of ethical care and to guide decisions about human care, health, death, daily life factors. It is a moral responsibility for nurses to learn about diverse ethical care practices in order to help clients retain their cultural values and ethical rights, and be cared for in therapeutic ways. The theory of culture care with focus on the worldview, social structure, and environmental context can help us discover ethical care in Western and non-Western cultures. And one of the most important discoveries in the study of ethical and moral values, norms, codes, covenants, principles, sanctions, rights, responsibilities, and obligations is to realize that these ethical aspects are *culturally constituted and expressed* within meaningful living contexts. While some progress is being made to discover comparative ethical care, much more work lies ahead. It will be encouraging to see nurses move forward to discover the universal and diverse dimensions of ethical human care.

# References

Aroskar, M. 1987. The interface of ethics and politics in nursing. *Nursing Outlook* 35(6): 268–72.

Beauchamp, T., and J. Childress. 1983. *Principles of biomedical ethics*, 2d ed. New York: Oxford University Press.

Boas, F. 1966. *Race, language and culture.* New York: Free Press.

Callahan, D. 1980. Autonomy: a moral good, not a moral obsession. *Hastings Center Report* 14(5): 40–42.

Carper, Barbara. 1979. The ethics of caring. *Advances in Nursing Science* 1(3): 11–19.

Curtin, L., and J. Flaherty. 1982. *Nursing ethics: Theories and Pragmatics.* Bowie, MD: Robert J. Brady Co.

Davis, A. J. 1981. Compassion, suffering, morality: Ethical dilemmas in caring. *Nursing law and ethics* 2(6): 8.

Downing, T., and G. Kushner. 1988. *Human rights and anthropology.* Cambridge, MA: Cultural Survival.

Fowler, M. 1986. Ethics without virtue. *Heart and Lung* 15(5): 528–30.

Fry, S. 1986. Moral decisions and ethical decisions in a constrained economic environment. *Nursing Economics* 4(4): 160–63.

Fry, S. 1988. The ethics of caring: Can it survive in nursing? *Nursing Outlook* 36(1): 48.

Gadow, S. 1980. *Existential advocacy—philosophical foundation for nursing.* San Francisco: Image Ideas Publication.

Gilligan, C. 1982. *In a different voice: Psychological theory and women's development.* Cambridge: Harvard University Press.

Haviland, W.A. 1987. *Cultural anthropology*, 5th ed. New York: Holt, Rinehart, and Winston.

Herskovits, M. 1964. *Cultural dynamics.* New York: Knopf.

Horn, B. 1978. Transcultural nursing and child-rearing of the Muckleshoot people. *Transcultural nursing: Concepts, theories and practices*, edited by M. M. Leininger, 223–39. New York: John Wiley and Sons.

Kluckhohn, C. 1970. *Mirror for man.* Greenwich, CT: Fawcett Press.

Lanham, Betty B. 1986. Ethics and moral precepts taught in schools of Japan and the United States. *Japanese culture and behavior: Selected readings*, edited by J. Libra and W. Libra, 280–96. Honolulu: University of Hawaii Press.

Leininger, M. 1970. *Nursing and anthropology: Two worlds to blend.* New York: John Wiley and Sons.

Leininger, M. 1974. Humanism, health and cultural values. *Health care dimensions: Health care issues*, 37–61. Philadelphia: F.A. Davis Co.

Leininger, M. 1978. *Transcultural nursing: Concepts, theories, and practices.* New York: John Wiley and Sons.

Leininger, M. 1983. Cultural care: An essential goal for nursing and health care. *American Association of Nephrology Nurses and Technicians* 10(5): 11–17.

Leininger, M. 1983–89. *Transcultural ethnonursing and ethnographic studies in urban community contexts.* Detroit: In press.

Leininger, M. 1984. *Care: The essence of nursing and health.* Thorofare, NJ: Charles B. Slack. Reprint 1988 by Wayne State University Press.

Leininger, M. 1985a. Transcultural care diversity and universality: A theory of nursing care. *Nursing and health care* 6(4): 202–12.

Leininger, M. 1985b. Ethnography and ethnonursing: Models and modes of qualitative data analysis. In *Qualitative research methods in nursing*, 33–73. Orlando, FL: Grune and Stratton.

Leininger, M. 1988a. Leininger's theory of nursing: Cultural care diversity and universality. *Nursing Science Quarterly* 1(4): 152–60.

Leininger, M. 1988b. *Care: Discovery and uses in clinical and community nursing.* Detroit: Wayne State University Press.

Leininger, M. 1989. The transcultural nurse specialist: Imperative in today's world. *Nursing and Health Care* 10(5): 251–56.

Luna, L. 1989. *Care and cultural context of Lebanese Muslims in an urban US community: An ethnographic and ethnonursing study conceptualized within Leininger's theory.* Ph.D. diss., Wayne State University.

MacIntyre, A. 1981. *After virtue.* Notre Dame, IN: University of Notre Dame Press.

Noddings, N. 1984. *Caring: A feminine approach to ethics and moral education.* Berkeley: University of California Press.

Ray, M. 1988. Discussion group summary: Ethical dilemmas in the clinical setting—time constraints, conflicts in interprofessional decision making. In *The ethics of care and the ethics of care: Synthesis in chronicity,* edited by J. Watson and D. Ray, 37–39. New York: National League for Nursing, Pub. #15-2237.

Ray, M. A. 1987. Health care economics and human caring in nursing: Why the moral conflict must be resolved. *Family Community Health* 10(1): 35–43.

Toulmin, S. 1987. The tyranny of principles. *Hastings Center Report* 11(6): 31–39.

Veach, R., and S. Fry. 1987. *Case studies in nursing ethics.* Philadelphia: J.B. Lyppincott.

Viens, D. 1989. A history of nursing's code of ethics. *Nursing Outlook* 37(1): 45–49.

Watson, J. 1985. *Nursing: Human science and human care. A theory of nursing.* Norwalk, CT: Appleton-Century-Crofts.

Watson, J., and M. Ray. 1988. *The ethics of care and the ethics of cure: Synthesis in chronicity.* New York: National League for Nursing, Pub. #15-2237.

Wenger, A. 1988. *The phenomenon of care in a high context culture: The old order Amish.* Ph.D. diss., Wayne State University.

# Respect and Caring: Ethics and Essence of Nursing

*Brighid Kelly, R.N., M.S., Ph.D.*

6

The purpose of this theoretical paper is to show respect and caring to be the ethics and essence of nursing. It is the author's position that if respect and caring are absent, nursing does not occur. The essential nature of respect and caring to the practice of nursing will be explicated initially by clarifying the concepts of respect and caring. Findings from a recent study in which informants provide an empirical definition of respect and caring provide the evidence for this thesis. Respect was defined by the informants as the message received by the other in initial interaction and described in terms of what the "ideal nurse" would do. Caring was perceived as multidimensional. It was described as "little things" and as having the dimensions of "taking time," showing love and concern, getting involved, being open and honest, being empathic and a good listener, being cheerful and friendly, and being a safe, competent nurse. The paper ends with a theoretical commentary on the relationship among the concepts of respect, caring, and nursing.

Respect for persons and caring are ideally integral to nursing practice. It remains puzzling, however, that these concepts are so noticeably absent from most theoretical descriptions of nursing. Nursing theorists have, for the most part, concentrated their attention on the roles of nurse and client, with little discussion of the ethical and moral dimensions inherent in the relationship. This has not always been the case, as many of our early nursing leaders including Florence Nightingale discussed the ethical role of nursing (Nutting 1916; Nightingale 1969). One explanation for the regrettable oversight is that, while nursing scholars reject the medical model and its influence on nursing, a review of knowledge development in nursing provides ample evidence of reductionism and empiricism. One may well conclude, as did Freire (1970), that oppressed groups, such as nurses, tend to emulate the values of the dominant group. In nursing, as in medicine, ethics and the broader concept of morals were typically classified under the category of metaphysics and consequently ignored. Thus, the scientific method and positivism became the dominant approach to inquiry in nursing.

Respect and caring are familiar concepts and thus may be taken for granted as found in nursing. Respect is an ethical concept, which is not only "the paramount moral attitude but all other moral principles are to be explained in terms of it" (Downie and Telfer 1970,2). One could easily spend a day browsing through books and articles on nursing ethics and never read more than a sentence or two on the concept of respect. On the other hand, the concept of caring has been well explicated philosophically and anthropologically (Leininger 1977; Watson 1979, 1985; Ray 1981; Gaut 1983; Bevis 1981). Recently a few empirical studies have surfaced in the nursing literature, which provide insight into the phenomenological experience of caring (Drew 1983; Gardner and Wheeler 1981; Reimen 1986). However, the view of caring as a nursing ethic is a relatively recent occurrence (Carper 1986; Fry 1988).

The purpose of this paper is to show that respect and caring are the ethics and the essence of nursing. It is the author's position that if respect and caring are absent, nursing does not occur. The essential nature of respect and caring to the practice of nursing will be explicated by initially clarifying the concepts of respect and caring. Empirical evidence, derived from a recent research study (B. Kelly 1987), will be provided to support respect and caring as the ethics of nursing. Finally, the paper will end with a theoretical commentary on the relationship among the concepts respect, caring, and nursing.

## Concept Clarification

*Respect for persons.* Downie and Telfer (1970, 87) describe the components of respect for persons as follows:

In so far as persons are thought of as self-determining agents who pursue objects of interest to themselves we respect them by showing active sympathy with them; in Kant's language, we make their ends our own. In so far as persons are thought of as rule-following we respect them by taking seriously the fact that the rules by which they guide their conduct constitute reasons for which may apply both to them and to ourselves. . . . These two components are independently necessary and jointly sufficient to constitute the attitude of respect which it is fitting to direct at persons.

Kant (1965), in distinguishing respect for persons from admiration or esteem, says respect for humanity is really respect for the moral law. Williams (1962, 159) says, "Each man [sic] is owed an effort at identification and not regarded as the surface to which a label can be applied." For the attributes of respect one can say that all persons are morally obligated to take seriously the values and goals of all other persons and in addition to be conscious that respect is not a reward for a particular behavior but is in fact a right.

*Caring.* Gaut (1983), in explicating a theoretical definition of caring, identified five conditions for "caring" to take place:

First condition: $S$ must be aware, either directly or indirectly, of the need for care in $X$.

Second condition: $S$ must know that certain things could be done to improve the situation.

Third condition: $S$ must intend to do something for $X$.

Fourth condition: $S$ must choose an action intended to serve as a means for bringing about a positive change in $X$, and then implement that action.

Fifth condition: The positive change in $X$ must be judged on the basis of what is good for $X$ rather than for $S$ or some other $Y$ or $Z$.

In briefly analyzing this view of caring one can say that Gaut believes that : (1) knowledge of the cared-for is necessary; (2) hope is necessary; (3) intention to act is necessary; (4) a "proper" action has been identified and implemented by the care-er; and (5) a judgment is made by the care-er that the positive change is what is good for the cared-for. What is not clear, however, is the role of the cared-for. Does X have a voice in the action intended to bring about "this positive change"? This raises the question of what part the cared-for plays in "caring."

Mayeroff (1971) identifies the major ingredients of caring as: knowing, patience, honesty, trust, humility, hope, and courage. He says that care-er and cared-for exist on the same level. They exist in equality. Noddings (1984) also refers to equality in the relationship between adults but also described how the cared-for may not be able, because of developmental maturity or other reasons, to respond as an equal to the care-er.

## Overview of the Study

The purpose of the study was to investigate, describe, and explain what senior baccalaureate nursing students internalize as professional values and to describe what they perceive as a commitment to professional ethics in nursing practice. The problem was explicated as a discrepancy between how nursing is expounded by the profession, particularly nursing educators, and how nursing is actually experienced by the general staff nurse. Since the aim of the study was to explore the experiences of the informants from their perspective, the qualitative method was chosen. Specifically, the design was a blend of inductive as described by Glaser and Strauss (1967) and deductive as outlined by Miles and Huberman (1983). The sample consisted of 23 senior baccalaureate nursing students of a total population of 120 who were in the final clinical rotation before graduation. Subjects were volunteers who gave informed consent, having been briefed on the purposes of the study and how their confidentiality would be protected. Data were collected in two ways: audiotaped, in-depth, open-ended interviews and written clinical logs. Content analysis was conducted on all data.

While a detailed description of data collection procedures and data analysis is beyond both the scope and the purpose of this paper, there is one element that had an important bearing on the findings. The bulk of data in this study was in response to the following statement: "I want you to think of nursing as you have experienced it and then tell me what you believe good nursing to be. I also want to know what you believe bad nursing to be. In other words what, in your experiences, are examples of nursing as you believe nursing ought be done and likewise examples of nursing as it ought not be done."

The study began as a study of ethics. Since the aim of the study was to have the informants express their views on professional values yet avoid an *a priori* fallacy, the investigator had each subject define the concept as it had meaning for him or her. The word *ethics* was not used in the early part of the interview because the investigator believed that the informants, being students, would become pre-occupied with providing the researcher with the "classroom" answer instead of their actual lived experiences. Each informant's data was classified under his or her code initials as either interview or log data and further organized by a coding system that identified the page number and the line number.

## The Findings

Results of the study revealed that informants perceived two concepts to be central to their view of "good" nursing, namely respect and caring. Data to support these concepts are presented in the informants' words.

*Respect.* The need to respect patients and families, self, colleagues, and the profession was identified as the most basic professional value. For example, respect for patients was described in terms of what the "ideal" nurse would do:

The first nurse was ideal. She came in and she listened to whatever the patient had to say to her. Even though she didn't understand it, she'd say "I didn't understand that please speak slower so that I can understand what you are saying to me." She was candid on the phone with the family. She gave her respect by pulling curtains when some procedure had to be done. She always explained from beginning to end. (N.O., interview, 2.20.)

Informants said respect was evidenced in the manner of interaction with the patient, i.e., listening, being honest, candid and "treating them like human beings." The importance of respect for these subjects was the message conveyed to the patient in the initial interaction, i.e., recognizing the patient as a person. However, these students were even more conscious of the need for respect when they perceived that it was absent. "The first thing that comes to mind . . . that really makes me angry is the nurses that don't listen to the patients. They go in the room and they want to hear a certain thing and no matter what the patient says that is the way they come out." (J.E., interview, 1.15.)

Another concern identified by these students was the manner in which patients were addressed: "Instead of calling the patients by their name, they—a lot of nurses—call the patients by their first name or they call them "honey." I work with a lot of older patients and I don't like that belittling. I think we should show respect. I wouldn't call my grandmother "honey"! I wouldn't call anyone older then me "honey." I hate it when people do it to me." (K.P. interview, 6.25.)

Respect for self, colleagues, and profession was described by most of the students in terms of self-respect as a professional, respect for colleagues, and "professional" behavior in general. Self-respect was described as assertiveness, continuing one's education, and promoting the rights of the nurse. Respect for colleagues was described in terms of collaborative, "professional" communications. Disrespect was evidenced by "backbiting" and lack of professional unity. Intra-professional respect was of considerable concern to these nursing students, as many perceived that nurses did not support each other. One subject said, "I don't think nurses are half as kind to each other as they are to the patient. I think there is a little lacking there that I wish were untrue . . . but I see a lot of backbiting of one another which is very distressing to me." (E.A., interview, 7.1.)

Respect for the profession was defined as striving for professionalization, subscribing to the professional values, and being involved in the professional organization. Disrespect for the profession was viewed as seeing nursing as a "job" rather than a career and not evidencing one's knowledge by assuming responsibility for decisions. Informant's were conscious of the need to be respected as professionals. Keeping standards high was viewed as a professional obligation, and students were aware of the constant need for vigilance in this area.

*Caring.* In analyzing informants' accounts, it was concluded that caring was closely aligned with respect in the minds of these subjects. In fact, the concepts were intertwined. The informants did not describe their experiences in terms of conceptual themes; it was the task of the investigator to separate and classify. In this case the investigator saw sufficient differences in the expression of these two concepts to separate them. The concepts of respect and caring were differentiated on the basis of conceptual quality. Caring was associated with showing "concern and love," providing psychological support, getting involved, being cheerful and friendly, and "taking the time" to do a good job. The concept of caring for these nursing students was best understood as all "the little things" as exemplified by the following: "It's the little things that are important to the patient—This man I had—he couldn't walk—he had been bedridden for a month—he couldn't even stand up and use his urinal. He needed help to walk and nurses didn't have the time to do it. Yet, there are nurses at the nurses' station just sitting and yakking. . . . Nurses need to have time to take care of patients." (K.P. interview, 15.25.) Another student said, "The exceptional nurses did those things, holding hands, talking to them, telling them what was going on. Being real open and honest with the families. Giving them psychological kind of support along with the physical." (F.V., interview, 1.11.)

The importance of the concept of caring for these nursing students was clearly evident. It would appear that they perceived caring as an essential ingredient to "good" nursing and as the "right" thing for a nurse to do. The pain of caring was another dimension expressed through the voices and experiences of these students. The dictionary defines caring as a state of mental suffering. To care is to be burdened, to be involved with someone. Noddings (1984) talks of caring as "engrossment." It would appear that caring is not easy. When one cares, one experiences pain as indicated from these findings:

I was terribly sad when I went in a room with one family whose 50-year-old daughter was the patient. She had lung cancer which had metastasized. They brought along a long page of questions which the doctor faithfully answered—the hardest one being the life expectancy which turned out to be only about six months with no treatment. I went out to try to comfort them. I felt so helpless. I ended up just simply staying with her for a while because she didn't want to talk. (L.T., log, 4.14.)

In the case of the young man dying on the unit now, the frustration and anger is very evident in their voices and the way they talk. As I said this is new to me. It is all very hard to sort through at times. The pain, the grief of the staff and the parents. The frustrations and helplessness felt when a kid is dying and you can't do anything. (H.G., log, 10.5.)

These findings reflect helplessness, underlying pain, and confusion as to the appropriateness or acceptability of these feelings: Am I supposed to feel this way? There also is an inference that nurses handle these feelings "in their own way."

In summary the results of the study revealed that the nursing students perceived respect and caring as the most basic professional values. Respect was empirically defined by these students as the message received by the other in initial interaction. It was described in terms of interactive demeanor, and the verbal and non-verbal message conveyed. Caring was perceived as multidimensional. It was described as "little things." It was empirically defined by these subjects as having the dimensions of "taking time," showing love and concern, getting involved, being open and honest, being empathic and a good listener, being cheerful and friendly, and being a safe, competent nurse. Caring was found to be painful and was described not only as subjects perceived it, but through their voices in experiencing it.

## Discussion

The significance of the findings may be obscured by their apparent simplicity and by the current emphasis on task completion and technical competence. Is that all there is to good nursing? The most signficant finding was that "good nursing" was perceived as an ethical concept. In other words, the students had integrated ethics into their concept of nursing.

Students' perception of caring as a nursing ethic was an unexpected finding. Although informants' familiarity with the concept of caring was in no small way related to their nursing education, the fact that they associated caring with ethics was interesting because this connection is not apparent in the nursing ethics literature. The recognition of caring as a moral duty has not been identified by nurse ethicists. Gilligan (1977) found that women's moral development centers around an ethic of care and a responsibility for not hurting others. According to Gilligan, the ethic of care becomes a universal obligation for women. Noddings (1984), in her feminist approach to ethics, describes the ethic of caring as "I must." She is, in many ways, advocating an ethic of virtue.

Although a few nursing scholars are beginning to discuss caring as an ethic (Carper 1986; Fry 1988; Watson 1988), the nursing ethics literature does not include caring as an ethic. Nurse ethicists are fairly consistent in their view of the guiding moral principles, which are usually identified as respect, beneficence, and justice. The ethical principles of autonomy and veracity tend to be incorporated under respect (Benjamin and Curtis 1982). The concept of caring is not included in the ANA *Code for Nurses* (1985). The word *care* appears once as in "health care." Moreover, in the ICN *Code for Nurses* (1973), although the term *care* appears four times, the concept of caring is not included. The question is, With so little connection between caring and ethics in the nursing ethics literature, why have the nursing students in this study made such a conceptual leap? Data from this study support that subjects believed a "good nurse" was a caring nurse. Therefore, it follows that in their minds caring and good nursing are one and the same. A logical conclusion would be that for these students ethical practice as caring is the essence of nursing.

# Theoretical Commentary

In qualitative research, theory should emerge from empirical data Patton says: "The cardinal principle of qualitative analysis is that causal relationships and theoretical statements be clearly emergent from and grounded in the phenomena studied. The theory emerges from the data; it is not imposed on the data" (1986, 278).

With these thoughts in mind, the following propositions form the basis of the theory emerging from the findings of this study. These propositions describe the relationship among the concepts respect, caring and nursing.

The practice of nursing is essentially moral in nature.

Respect for persons and caring are the ethics of nursing.

Respect, as a nursing ethic, is evidenced by respect for clients and families, self, colleagues, and the profession.

Caring, as a nursing ethic, is evidenced by caring for clients and families, self, colleagues, and the professions.

Respect and caring are necessary but not sufficient elements of nursing.

Respect precedes caring in the nurse-client relationship.

In the absence of respect, caring cannot take place.

In the absence of caring, nursing does not take place.

## Proposition 1: The practice of nursing is essentially moral in nature.

Silva (1983) described nursing as a duty, a moral art, and an autonomous profession. Her thesis is that nursing owes society a duty to care because society and nursing have a social contract. She describes the moral art of nursing as taking care of patients by touching, teaching, comforting, listening, diminishing, suffering, and generally doing for persons what they cannot do for themselves. Nightingale saw nursing in her own life as a "call from God" (Woodham-Smith 1983). On May 29, 1900, she wrote the following letter to her probationers at St. Thomas' Hospital:

My dear children:
You have called me you Mother-Chief. It is an honour to me and a great honour to call you my children. Always keep up the honour of this honourable profession. . . . We dishonour [it] when we are bad or careless nurses, we dishonour [it] when we do not do our best to relieve suffering even in the meanest creature. (Schuyler 1975, 166)

That statement by Nightingale supports the notion that nursing is essentially a moral activity. Prior to the influence of Nightingale, nursing was provided by religious orders because ministering to the sick was viewed as the essence of moral obligation. The history of American nursing is replete with examples of women who risked everything to focus their lives on service to others (Kalisch and Kalisch 1986). Ministering to the needs of others is the essence of nursing.

## Proposition 2: Respect for persons and caring are the essential ethics of nursing.

This statement was supported by data in this study, but there is much wider support for such a proposition.

Respect. The first ethical injunction of the *Code for Nurses* speaks to the provision of respect for all humans. The ethics of nursing refers to the conduct of nurses while they are nursing and to the motives and ends of their professional decision making. L. Kelly (1975, 208) says, "The true ethical core of all professional codes derives from the rights and dignity of the individual—treating the patient as a person." Curtin (Curtin and Flaherty 1982, 3) has consistently stated that ethics in nursing is more evidenced by the day-to-day activities among nurses and patients than "fabulous life and death issues."

*Caring.* The connection between caring and ethics was made by Gilligan (1977). She described a model of moral development for females based on caring. Gilligan believes that females have had to develop a sense of responsibility based on the universal principle of caring in order to survive. Noddings (1984), an educationist, also proposes a feminine view of ethics based on caring. Her argument is that the basis of all moral action is the memory of being cared for. Her belief is that all moral decisions are grounded in natural caring. This view of ethics is similar to the psychological view that one needs to be loved in order to love. Montagu (1975, 2) says, "She knows how to love, for the only way one learns to love is by being loved." This leads one to conclude that caring is taught by example. The implications are clear for nursing instructors whose clients are nursing students.

Are nurses ethically obligated to "care" for their clients? Before answering this question one must be clear on the meaning ascribed to *care* in this context. Leininger (1981) has studied and identified the essential characteristics present in care such as comfort, compassion, concern, empathy, enabling, involvement, and facilitating. Caring is philosophically defined as being concerned, involved, having an active sympathy, which manifests itself in supporting the cared-for's goals for growth, and self-actualization (Ray 1981). It may be equated with being concerned about someone or charged with the protection of a person. The idea that "caring" involves some element of personal giving of oneself or sacrifice has also been discussed by philosophers. Downie and Telfer (1970) describe this as an "active sympathy" with others and call it *agape*. May (1969) says the opposite of caring is apathy or indifference. The answer to the above question is a resounding "yes". Nurses are ethically obligated to "care" for their clients.

## Proposition 3: Respect, as a nursing ethic, is evidenced by respect for clients and families respect for self, colleagues, and the nursing profession.

Since respect for clients and families has been discussed above, a brief clarification of the concept of self-respect is in order as viewed by several philosophers and analyzed in relation to the findings. Kant's views on self-respect are found in *The Doctrine of Virtue* (1964, 434): [A person] possesses, in other words, a dignity (an absolute inner worth) by which he [sic] expects respect for himself from all other rational beings in the world." In discussing one's duties to oneself, Kant lists vices one should avoid, that is, vices that degrade one's moral being. Among these are servility, avarice, and lying. Although Kant discusses self-deception at length, he says that no violation of a person's duty to self is worse than dishonesty. Downie and Telfer (1970, 87) believe that self-respect involves being one's own master and being self-determining. Hill (1982) believes that self-respect is when the person has personal standards or ideals and believes that he (or she) lives by them. Sachs (1982), in analyzing whether self-respect and respect for others are independent, concludes that persons deficient in self-respect are "sorely lacking" in respect for others.

The informants in this study provided evidence of how nurses ought to respect colleagues and the profession. They identified the need to see oneself as professional, to act in a professional manner toward one's colleagues, to continue one's education, to strive for unity among nurses, and to be active in one's professional organization. Collegiality was perceived as manifested by respect for others' knowledge and the sharing of ideas through networking and professional cooperation. Respect for the profession entailed not merely viewing nursing as a profession, but acceptance of the professional values of professional growth and a commitment to the professional code.

## Proposition 4: Caring as an ethic in nursing is evidenced by caring for clients and families, self, colleagues, and the profession.

Caring for clients and families has been discussed above. Caring for self, colleagues, and the profession is ideally integral to a caring profession. Kelsey (1981) says that caring for self involves listening to ourselves and forgiving ourselves. Healthy persons know themselves and exhibit trust and confidence in their own ability to deal with situations when they come along, says Tubesing (1983). He also says that self-care involves practicing self-disclosure, reflection, developing healthy relationships, and nurturing support groups.

Caring for colleagues was described by informants as involvement and support in professional relationships. Mayeroff (1971, 3) states: "caring is helping others to grow and to actualize themselves." With regard to manifesting caring toward the profession ANA *Code of Ethics* specifies that nurses have an ethical obligation to contribute to the development of the profession's body of knowledge, to participate in the profession's efforts to implement and improve standards of care, and to participate in efforts to improve standards of employment conducive to high-quality nursing care. These are the goals of the nursing profession, and nurses who participate in any or all of these efforts are demonstrating a "caring" attitude to the profession.

## Proposition 5: Respect and caring are necessary but not sufficient elements of nursing.

Respect and caring are essential elements of nursing, but these properties alone are not enough. Professional status is not determined by merely subscribing to the values of a profession. Nightingale said, "Nature has laws or conditions for health and for sickness as for everything else. We have to learn them." (Schuyler, 1975, 165)

The nursing students in this study identified their educational program as the most influential force in shaping their view of themselves as nurses. Many students also made reference to the baccalaureate as the minimum educational qualification for entry into the profession. In the absence of knowledge, respect and caring are insufficient for nursing to take place.

## Proposition 6: Respect for persons precedes caring in the nurse-client relationship.

The findings of this study confirm the primary nature of respect. Kant claimed that every human being was an end in himself [sic] and therefore worthy of respect, and he distinguished persons from things in asserting that "respect always applies to persons, never to things." According to Hill (1982, 129), a philosopher, basic respect as a human being does not have to be earned. Humans need not participate in order to be respected. One can, therefore, respect another human being without knowing him or her. On the other hand, caring cannot take place without knowledge. To illustrate this concept one might recall a moving scene in the film *The Elephant Man* (1980, directed by David Lynch). The "creature" is being chased by a mob through the London underground and when cornered, cries out in desperation, "I am not an animal, I am a man." As the story unfolds, one is struck by the way in which the "creature" is treated when it is discovered that not only is he not an imbecile, he is brilliant. He is then addressed as "Mr. John Merrick" and held in high esteem. In examining the doctor's attitude, one deduces that the doctor respected "the creature" from the beginning because of his humanity, but it was only when he began to know John that a caring relationship was evident.

## Proposition 7: In the absence of respect, caring cannot take place.

The essence of caring is wishing a person well—wanting what is best for him or her. This attitude is logically impossible in the absence of respect. Mayeroff (1971) believes that respect is primary in a caring relationship and says a person needs to be viewed as an individual and not "used" by the care-er. He provides the example of a father caring for his child. Instead of dominating and wanting to possess the other, the father wants the child to grow in his or her own right.

## Proposition 8: In the absence of caring, nursing does not take place.

Caring as the essence of nursing has been discussed by several nursing leaders (Leininger 1977; Watson 1979; Ray 1981; Boyle 1981). Carper says: "This basic dictum to be compassionate, humane and caring toward those for whom we provide care is most often expressed in the phrase 'treat the person not merely the patient.' To be concerned with the 'whole person' and to practice with consideration and sensitivity for the integrity of the human self is basically an ethical injunction" (1986, 1).

According to Leininger (1981), caring is the central and unifying focus for the body and practice of nursing. Ray (1981) says caring is perceived as involving a process of co-presence, giving, receiving, communication, and in essence loving. Bevis (1981) says concern is the closest to being synonymous with caring and compares it to Tillich's use of the term *ultimate concern*. Although Bevis does not use the term *duty*, she says *caring* is a force, a compelling action. Watson (1979), in explicating ten carative factors integral to the nurse-client relationship, says that focusing on feelings promotes self-awareness in the nurse and thus is conducive to acceptance of client's feelings—both positive and negative. She says nursing is the science of caring.

The ANA social policy statement (1980) describes the nature of nursing as interactive and says that nursing has historically focused on nurturing and creating a physiologic, psychologic, and sociocultural environment in which the patient (and family) can gain or maintain health. The students in this study valued caring as the essence of nursing for them. In fact, when they were asked to identify the one value so important to them that they could not practice nursing without it, more of them identified caring than any other value. Ozar (1987) speaks of the fundamental values and principles of the nursing profession. He says that in order to truly be a nurse, one needs to have a wholehearted commitment to the principles and values of the profession. He goes on to say that one who enters with reservations about these values and principles cannot be viewed as a full member of the nursing profession. A logical inference from this statement is that a person who does not practice according to the values and principles of nursing is not practicing nursing. In the absence of caring, nursing does not take place.

## Summary

The findings of this study and the emergent theory together provide a tapestry of nursing. First, nursing is a caring ministry. Second, nursing requires a specialized body of knowledge. Third, nursing respects the uniqueness and wholeness of all persons. And fourth, nursing recognizes and respects the nurse's role in manipulating environmental forces. These assumptions and beliefs about nursing are stated in terms of the ideal, i.e., what nursing ought to be. One could make a case for the notion that the results of this study more accurately reflect the reality of nursing.

The thesis of this paper is that ethical decision making is central to every nursing act. Decision making grounded in ethics is not a particular mode of reasoning to which one refers in certain situations. It is an element of nursing. The nursing students in this study perceived that ethical nursing was evidenced in ordinary, everyday nurse-patient interactions and in collegial relationships. Levine said: "Ethical behavior is not the display of one's moral rectitude in times of crises. It is the day-by-day expression of one's commitment to other persons and the ways in which human beings relate to one another in their daily interactions" (1977, 847).

# References

American Nurses' Association, 1980. *Nursing: A social policy statement.* Kansas City, MO: American Nurses' Association.

American Nurses' Association. 1985. *Code for nurses with interpretative statements.* Kansas City, MO: American Nurses' Association.

Benjamin, M., and J. Curtis. 1982. *Ethics in nursing.* New York: Oxford University Press.

Bevis, E. 1981. Caring: A life force. In *Caring: An essential human need,* edited by M. Leininger. Thorofare, NJ: Charles B. Slack.

Boyle, J. 1981. An application of the structure-functional method of the phenomenon of caring. In *Caring: An essential human need,* edited by M. Leininger. Thorofare, NJ: Charles B. Slack.

Carper, B. 1986. The ethics of caring. In *Ethical issues in nursing,* Rockville, MD: Aspen Systems Corp.

Curtin, L., and M. J. Flaherty. 1982. *Nursing ethics: Theories and pragmatics.* Bowie, MD: Robert J. Brady Co.

Drew, N. 1983. Exclusion and confirmation. A phenomenology of patients experiences with caregivers. *Image* 18(2): 39–43.

Downie, R. S., and E. Telfer. 1970. *Respect for persons.* New York: Schocken Books.

Freire, P. 1982. *Pedagogy of the oppressed.* New York: Continuum Publishing.

Fry, S. 1988. The ethic of caring: Can it survive in nursing? *Nursing Outlook* 36(1): 48.

Gardner, F., and E. Wheeler. E. 1981. Patients and staff perceptions of supportive nursing behaviors. In *Caring: An essential human need,* edited by M. Leininger. Thorofare, NJ: Charles B. Slack.

Gaut, D. 1983. Development of a theoretically adequate description of caring. *Western Journal of Nursing Research* 5(4): 313–24.

Gilligan, C. 1977. In a different voice: Women's conception of self and morality. *Harvard Educational Review* 47: 481–517.

Glaser, B., and A. Strauss. 1967. *The discovery of grounded theory.* Chicago: Aldine.

Hill, T. 1982. Self-respect reconsidered. In *Respect for persons,* edited by O. H. Green, New Orleans: Tulane University Press.

International Council of Nurses. 1973. *The code for nurses.* Geneva, Switzerland.

Kalisch, P., and B. Kalisch. 1986. *The advance of American nursing.* Boston: Little, Brown.

Kant, I. 1964. *The doctrine of virtue,* translated by McGregor. New York: Harper and Row.

Kant, I. 1965. *The metaphysics of morals,* translated by J. Ladd. Indianapolis: Bobbs-Merrill Co.

Kelly, B. 1987. *Perception of professional ethics among senior baccalaureate nursing students.* Ph.D. diss., Ohio State University.

Kelly, L. 1975. *Dimensions of professional nursing.* New York: Macmillan.

Kelsey, M. 1981. *Caring.* Ramsey, NJ: Paulist Press.

Leininger, M. 1977. Caring: The essence and central focus of nursing. *American Nurses' Foundation Nursing Research Reports.* 12(1): 2–14.

Leininger, M. 1981. *Caring: An essential human need.* Thorofare, NJ: Charles B. Slack. Reprint 1988 by Wayne State University Press.

Levine, M. 1977. Nursing ethics and the ethical nurse. *American Journal of Nursing* 77(5): 846–47.

May, R. (1969). *Love and will.* New York: Norton.

Mayeroff, M. 1971. *On caring.* New York: Harper and Row.

Miles, M., and A. Huberman. 1983. *Qualitative data analysis.* Beverly Hills, CA: Sage Publications.

Montagu, A. 1975. *The practice of love.* Englewood Cliffs, NJ: Prentice Hall.

Noddings, N. 1984. *Caring: A feminine approach to ethics and moral education.* Berkeley: University of California Press.

Nightingale, F. 1969. *Notes on nursing: What it is and what it is not.* New York: Dover Publications.

Nutting, A. 1916. Some ideals in training school work. *Annual Report.* New York: National League of Nursing Education.

Ozar, D. 1987. The demands of professions and their limits. In *The professional commitment*, edited by Quinn and Smith. Philadelphia: W.B. Saunders.

Patton, M.Q. 1986. *Qualitative evaluation methods.* Beverly Hills, CA: Sage Publications.

Ray, M. 1981. A philosophical analysis of caring within nursing. In *Caring: An essential human need*, edited by M. Leininger. Thorofare, NJ: Charles B. Slack.

Reimen, D. 1986. The essential structure of caring interaction: Doing phenomenology. Munhill, *Nursing research: A qualitative respective*, edited by Munhall and Oiler. Norwalk, CT.: Appleton Century Croft.

Sachs, D. 1982. Self, respect and respect for others: Are they independent. *Respect for persons*, edited by O.H. Green, New Orleans: Tulane University Press. 100–128.

Schuyler C. 1975. *Molders of modern nursing: Florence Nightingale and Louisa Schuyler* Ann Arbor, MI: University Microfilms International.

Silva, M. 1983. The American Nurses' Association's position on nursing and social policy. *Journal of Advanced Nursing* 8(2): 147–51.

Tubesing, D. 1983. *The caring question.* Minneapolis: Augsburg Publishing.

Watson, J. 1979. *Nursing: The philosophy and science of caring.* Boston: Little, Brown.

Watson, J. 1985. *Nursing: Human science and human care. A theory of nursing.* Norwalk, CT: Appleton-Century-Crofts

Watson, J. 1988. New dimensions of human caring theory. *Nursing Science Quarterly* 1(4): 175–81.

Williams, B. 1962. The idea of equality. In *Philosophy, Politics and Society*, edited by Laslett and Runceman. New York: Barnes and Noble.

Woodham-Smith, C. 1983. *Florence Nightingale 1820–1910.* New York: Atheneum.

# Noddings's Caring and Public Policy: A Linkage and Its Nursing Implications

*Phyllis R. Schultz, R.N., Ph.D., and Robert C. Schultz, Ph.D.*

7

Nell Noddings, in *Caring: A Feminine Approach to Ethics and Moral Education* (1984), can be interpreted as proposing to reduce ethics to personal feelings, such as the "longing for goodness" in one-to-one and other intimate human relationships. But the work of forming public policy (including health policy) seems to call for impersonal rules and criteria to justify rational choices affecting communities, populations, and more-or-less global political units. Is an ethic of caring, then, irrelevant to large-scale policy formation? And, if so, is Noddings's "feminine approach" out of place where nurses focus on such macro-entities in their practice, theory development, and research?

The purpose of this inquiry, which begins from a sympathetic critique of Noddings's intimate ethics of caring, is to link caring to the ethical aspects of policy-making. The conclusion is that the notion of "moral community" provides the needed linkage between the ethics of caring and the ethics of public policy-making. Some implications for nursing are that : (1) the concept of professionalism cannot properly be separated from that of community; (2) the "client" for nursing will often be a plurality of persons, an organization and/or a community; (3) the practice of a caring nurse will frequently have to take the form of political action.

This inquiry is a conversation between nursing theory and moral philosophy. Ultimately, the conversation is about the idea of moral community and about using this idea to inform nursing theory. Our argument runs as follows: In setting forth a feminist-oriented ethics of caring, Nell Noddings (1984) has offered a refreshing corrective to the Enlightenment legacy of rule-ethics. But an adequate ethical theory ought to encompass the domain of public policy and law, in addition to the domain of intimate relationships stressed by Noddings. The idea of moral community, with its stress on personal virtue, offers a link between the norms of caring-between-intimates and the norms needed to guide programs, policies, and laws in the wider public domain. And this communitarian perspective supports the expansion of nursing theory to recognize nurse administrators, community health nurses, and even nurse-politicians, as practitioners understood to be caring for clients.

The ethics of rules, as used in this inquiry, matured in the eighteenth and early nineteenth centuries in the work of Kant in Germany and the Utilitarians in Britain (Kant [1785] 1948; Bentham 1789; Mill 1863). These writers expressed the demand

---

The original version of this paper was presented by the authors in dialogue format at the Ninth National Caring Conference, "Ethics and Morality of Caring," Menlo Park, CA, April 26–28, 1987.

of Europe's new middle classes for equal rights and the rule of law. Their work also reflects the aspiration to apply scientific rationality to the governance of human society. We may reasonably imagine, of course, that much interpersonal caring had occurred in earlier, medieval society, just as it surely did later, in this country, on the plantations of the antebellum South. But interpersonal caring, whether from noblesse oblige or Christian charity, is not enough to counteract what some, more recent writers have termed "socially unnecessary domination" (Haberman 1975). To counter social domination, ethical rules were formulated, that served as constraints on hurtful and unfair conduct and as guides for the nonviolent resolution of conflict. The problem with such rules, however, is that, while they embody basic democratic ideals, they are often applied in uncaring, dehumanizing, and destructive ways. This last fact is a major point of departure in Noddings's account of ethics.

## The Nursing Theory Problem

Noddings's account of the ethical has struck a responsive chord in nurses because it seems to articulate much of what the practice and the discipline is about. At the same time, its lack of a policy dimension has a counterpart in current nursing theory. First, the currently accepted concepts and assumptions in nursing perpetuate a view that health is a phenomenon of *individual* persons, and that response to actual and potential health problems is a result of *individual* human agency. This view neglects the impact of the social, political, and economic determinants of health, and it neglects the role of collective agencies in solving health problems or enhancing health. As a field of inquiry, nursing suffers from what has been called "ontological individualism . . . the belief that the individual has a primary reality whereas society is a second-order, derived or artificial construct" (Bellah) et al. 1985, 334). A corollary of this first point is that caring is the result of a nurse's individual human agency and is, therefore, essentially an interpersonal phenomenon.

In actual nursing practice, however, community health nurses and nurse administrators define the client they care for as "more than one" (Schultz 1987). Caring is experienced as being present to and engaged with a group, or as implementing a "spirit of democratic 'active participation' with a community" (Goeppinger 1984, 403). Thus there is a "lack of fit" between existing nursing theory and the actual practice of nurses in specialty areas in which corporate or public policy is a part of the praxis of the discipline. To correct this limitation, nursing theory must be developed that identifies organizations, communities, and pluralities or persons as appropriately defined "clients," that is, as appropriate beneficiaries of caring. And caring and the ethics of caring must be extended beyond the interpersonal for nursing to influence public policy from its unique "caring" perspective. Before such extensions can be elaborated, however, key features of Noddings's feminist ethics should be reviewed.

## Noddings's Account of Ethics and Its Limitations

Nell Noddings's book is a refreshing corrective to many years of moral philosophizing. Part of what is refreshing about this book is seeing its author shine through the writing, as a living source and exemplar of the theory she offers to her readers. Her theory is enriched by personal examples and provocative stories. Her human warmth, coupled with tough-minded common sense, leaves the reader confident of the happy fate of those who dwell in, and pass through, the Nodding's kitchen and garden. But there are also general theses to be attended to here—one positive and constructive, the other negative and rejecting.

The positive thesis is that ethics has its origins and its development in interpersonal caring. Caring for another is being receptive and responsive to a "cared-for" person. Caring is a natural way to relate to another, a way best expressed in many cultural traditions by mothers. When natural caring encounters obstacles, the remembered experience of having been cared for oneself motivates the "one-caring" to abide by the ethical "I must." This acceptance expresses one's longing for the good of the other and, at the same time, enhances one's own ethical ideal. At its best, this way of being toward others creates and sustains joy.

The negative thesis in Noddings's account is that ethics understood as rules and reasoning, as the quest for justified, universalizable judgments, "simply cannot be broadly applied in the actual world" (1984, 3). In the name of rules and principles, we take pride in fighting and killing one another. Rules "require a move to abstraction that tends to destroy the uniqueness of the caring itself" (33). Rules are "destructive" (47), and when we encounter rules embodied in institutions, "many of us have been reduced to cases by the very machinery that has been instituted to care for us" (66).

Admittedly, there are some hints in Noddings—in her language of "chains of caring"—that suggest a broader view, one that extends caring beyond the "cared-for" who is "here with me." But these remain mainly hints. For the most part, Noddings's account of ethics is limited to a celebration of caring among intimates. And what is left out are the larger domains where human actions, guided by policy and law, often significantly affect other persons. Where are the ethical ideals and constraints—such as liberty and equality—of our nation's founders? Where are the ethical prescriptions and limitations for our conduct as global citizens such as in the Universal Declaration of Human Rights? In these larger political domains, and in the organizations of business, education, and health care, we need an ethics that guides the creators and maintainers of these non-intimate agencies of human interaction.

To extend Noddings's account, as proposed in this paper, will require recognizing the constraining role of ethics, as in Aristotle's view that some acts are just plain wrong (Aristotle 1985). The extension will also accept the mandate of Jesus in the parable of the Good Samaritan to treat the suffering stranger as "my neighbor." Furthermore, the extension will recognize that rational justification, which Noddings so explicitly rejects, has a positive role to play in human affairs. True, justification often amounts to little more than a bureaucratic weapon to back up uncaring treatment or no treatment at all; or it's used simply to protect against litigation. But if rationality is understood as constructive dialectic, embodying equality and respect for persons, it becomes a friend, not an enemy of caring.

## Extending the Definition of the "One-Cared For": Conditions for Sustaining the Ethical Ideal

By confining the ethics of caring to the interpersonal, Noddings fails to acknowledge that the norms and structures of the society and its institutions either support and sustain the ethical ideal of individuals or diminish it. These norms and structures are formulated, in part, by corporate and public policy. So how can a link be forged between Noddings's account of caring and the ethics embedded in policy? Extending the definition of key concepts in her thesis and emphasizing others may help. For example, the "one-cared-for" can be extended to include a plurality of persons. Also, explicating how a "relation" can be actualized with pluralities may be helpful. Also, clarifying the concept of caring itself is also critical, and here it may be helpful to complement Noddings's key concepts with Gaut's three conditions of a theoretically adequate definition of caring (Gaut 1983). First, the one-caring must have knowledge of $X$, which means knowledge of the one/ones-cared-for. Second, the one-caring must choose and implement action based on knowledge and intend to bring about a positive change in the one/ones-cared-for. Third, the "positive change condition must be judged solely on the basis of a 'welfare-of-$X$' criterion" (Gaut 1983, 322).

Consider, as an example, the practice of a maternal-child nursing consultant in a state health department. Let us assume that the "other" is a plurality of pregnant women without access to prenatal care. The consultant has knowledge about pregnant women in need of prenatal care and knows that the design and implementation of a program of access to this type of care could improve their situation. The consultant chooses and implements action, that is, she designs a program, writes rules of eligibility, outlines procedures for implementing the program, writes a grant request for funding, and supervises the implementation of the program. These activities are carried out with the intention that the action will bring about a positive change in the "ones-cared-for." Through access to and receipt of prenatal care, the women enhance their chances for healthy babies and healthy selves. The positive change in the "ones-cared-for" is not based on chance, whim, the self-interest of the consultant, or the cost-savings objectives of some other individual or agency. Rather, the positive change is based solely on the criterion of the "welfare-of-those-cared-for." It is for their own welfare and that of their unborn children than the pregnant women receive prenatal care—the result of the caring action of the consultant. When the community health nursing consultant observes, whether by personal observation or by written reports, that the ones cared for are responding, the "circle of relation" is completed, thus sustaining the consultant's ethical ideal. The linkage forged in this example illustrates the features of the program that (1) satisfy both Noddings's account and Gaut's conditions of caring, and (2) suggest how rules and policy provide the framework for action that sustains the ethical ideal.

## The Linkage Between Caring and Policy Ethics

In the above example, it is *assumed* that ethics applies to the direct interpersonal rendering of caring to particular pregnant women—to "Pam" and "Laura" and

"Kathy." But what is *asserted* here, in addition, is that the ethics of caring also applies to the conceiving of the program of care, to politicking for it, to researching and planning and institutionalizing it. This assertion implies, in turn, that ethics must encompass rules such as "it's wrong to deny services on the basis of inability to pay, or race, or sexual orientation." And ethics must also include (*pace* Noddings) admittedly abstract virtues like fairmindedness, courage, perseverance, and honesty.

Thus, the above assertions lead to the following question: What sort of ethics provides theoretical space for *both* the intimate domain of interpersonal caring *and* the rest of the social order—the social order that is large in population, complex in structure, freedom loving and egalitarian in aspiration, and laced with conflicts that require nonviolent resolution?

A.C. MacIntyre, in *After Virtue* (1984), has made a major contribution to the communitarian perspective in his recent attempt to "dust off" the ethics of Aristotle. In MacIntyre's account, as in Aristotle's, the primary focus of ethics lies in virtues, those qualities of personal character that make social life possible and good. This focus on persons instead of rules is somewhat like Noddings's feminine approach; however, here the virtues are grounded less in individual impulses to care for another person and more in social practices. These practices are what constitute human existence nearly everywhere—the practices of homemaking, of organizing political action, of providing for education, health care, and national security. And the exercise of personal virtues—honesty, fairmindedness, and the rest—is essential for the success of such universal practices.

While not occupying the central place in ethics, rules are nonetheless essential for setting basic limits on the conduct of members of the community. As Aristotle put it, while virtue normally involves finding the mean between excess and deficiency in action, there is just no acceptable place in society for adultery, murder, and certain other actions—they are ruled out! And the conformity to such rules provides a sort of moral space within which individuals can nurture and express what Noddings calls their "ethical ideals." A case in point is that of the community health nurse and her rule-governed program of prenatal care.

Finally, persons, central in the communitarian perspective, are recognized as being constituted by relations, as having unique "stories," as being embedded in evolving social traditions, as initiated into practices embodying excellence, and as having both instrumental and intrinsic worth (MacIntyre 1984, chapters 14 and 15). Furthermore, the communitarian perspective proposed here recognizes that organizations and communities have narratives and traditions that embody practices of excellence. Such insitutionalized practices, like the individuals who participate in them, have both instrumental and intrinsic worth.

## Implications for Nursing of the Communitarian Perspective

Public policy, then, inspired by Noddings's ethics of caring, extended by communitarian virtue ethics, and informed by the discipline of nursing, would display several features. It would: (1) clearly reflect the valuing of humans as "persons," that is, the language of policy would avoid reducing individuals or groups to more objects or economic units of service consumption; (2) foster self-initiative and personal and community empowerment, such that the persons affected could engage in "the free pursuit of their projects" (Noddings 1984, 81); and (3) be changed if, in its implementation, the policy made interpersonal caring, or engagement with the plurality, difficult or impossible, thereby diminishing the ethical ideals of all those involved.

To realize nursing's potential contribution to public policy, several challenges must be met. First, nursing theory must be developed that explicitly reflects pluralities of persons and interactional units such as organizations, corporations, communities, nation-states, and the world. Second, nursing's knowledge from research and practice must be recognized as constituting a basis for expertise in policy analysis and formulation, and policy-making activity must be recognized as a legitimate practice of the nursing profession. Third, there is a need to gather case examples of how corporate and public policies either sustain or diminish the ethical ideal of clients and nurses. Beyond these challenges, however, lies perhaps the greatest challenge of communitarian virtue ethics to nurses, a challenge that goes beyond the development of the discipline's theoretical foundations and the exemplification of its expertise. This challenge is to socialize and educate all nursing practitioners to have the courage, honesty, generosity, fairmindedness, and perseverance to assert the intrinsic value of caring and to demand that society recognize this value through the fair allocation of resources for its support.

Finally, it must be emphasized that Noddings's formulation of the ethics of caring is not rejected in this paper. Rather, its definition as only interpersonal is held to be too narrow. Nurses are urged to expand their vision by extending the definitions of their disciplinary concepts and adopting a communitarian ethics. Such an ethics would combine a feminine core with frameworks of minimal rules and with personal virtues that connect core and frameworks in a new, broadly conceived vision of professional nursing practice.

# References

Aristotle. 1985. *Nichomachean ethics*, translated by T. Irwin. Indianapolis: Hackett Publishing.

Bellah, R.N., et al. 1985. *Habits of the heart: Individualism and commitment in American Life*. Berkeley: University of California Press.

Bentham, J. 1789. *Introduction to the principles of morals and legislation*. Oxford: Oxford University Press.

Gaut, D. 1983. Development of a theoretically adequate description of caring. *Western Journal of Nursing Research* 5(4):313–24.

Goeppinger, J. 1984. Community as client: Using the nursing process to promote health. In *Community health nursing: Process and practice for promoting health*, edited by M. Stanhope and J. Lancaster, 317–404. St. Louis: C.V. Mosby.

Habermas, J. 1975. *Legitimation crisis*, translated by T. McCarthy. Boston: Beacon Press.

Kant, I. (1785) 1948. *Law, or Kant's groundwork of the metaphysic of morals*, translated by J.J. Patton. London.

MacIntyre, A.C. 1984. *After virtue: A study in moral theory*, 2d ed. Notre Dame, IN: University of Notre Dame Press.

Mill, J.S. (1863). *Utilitarianism.* London.

Noddings, N. 1984. *Caring: A feminine approach to ethics and moral education.* Berkeley: University of California Press.

Schultz, P.R. 1987. When client is more than one: Extending the foundational concept of person. *Advances in Nursing Science* 10(1):72–86.

# The Virtue of Caring in Nursing

*Virginia Knowlden, R.N., M.A. Ed.D.*

8

This chapter explicates caring as a virtue in the practice of professional nurses in community health care. The theoretical framework concerning virtue was drawn from the writings of Crossin (1985), Hauerwas (1974), and MacIntyre (1981). The data was derived from secondary analysis of the recorded verbatim data of twenty female professional nurses' practices and thirty patients from the author's research, "The Meaning of Caring in the Nurse's Role" (Knowlden 1985). Following MacIntyre's (1981) indication, three stages were identified for caring to be a virtue. Secondary analysis indicated that caring is made apparent in nursing practice as a virtue through stories of actions and attitudes that reflect the deep knowledge nurses have of themselves as committed caregivers.

This paper will explain the virtue of caring in nursing as revealed in nurses' practices. The author draws substance from a secondary analysis of the raw data from the study "The Meaning of Caring in the Nursing Role" (Knowlden 1985), and uses its theory from the works of MacIntyre (1981) and Hauerwas (1974), which concern virtue.

According to Webster, virtue means a "conformity to a standard of what is right and good" (1974, 1307). Erikson defines virtue as "certain human qualities of strength" (1964, 113). Virtue is a quality of human excellence, a trait that a person may possess or aspire to. Moral virtue is an acquired habit or disposition to do what is morally right or praiseworthy, to act in accordance with morals, principles, ideals, or rules (Beauchamp and Childress 1983, 264). Gaffney (1979) indicates that virtue is a theory or system of moral values. Virtue differs from ethics in that the possession of virtue enables us to exercise choice in order to achieve a purpose. Ethics is the discipline dealing with what is good or evil, right or wrong. Ethics serves in an advisory capacity, suggesting arguments and considerations.

Virtue is of two types: the theological and the cardinal. Theological virtue consists of faith, hope, and love; cardinal virtues consist of prudence, temperance, courage, and justice. These qualities of human excellence are often taken "for granted as basic, indispensable ingredients of a humanly good life" (Gaffney 1979, 98).

Crossin (1985) suggests that virtues are strengths acquired developmentally. Hope, will, purpose, and competence are virtues developed in childhood; fidelity in adolescence; and love, care, and wisdom in adulthood. According to Erikson, "care is the widening concern for what has been generated by love, necessity, or accident;

it overcomes the ambivalence adhering to irreversible obligation" (Crossin 1985, 72). Caring is linked to virtue through its relationship to love particularly and to the other virtues as well, especially courage and hope. Care can extend to a person's works and ideas as well as to children (Mayeroff 1971).

In order to explain a virtue, it is necessary to accept "some prior account of certain features of social and moral life in terms of which the virtue has to be defined and explained" (MacIntyre 1981, 74). The virtue of caring in nursing emerges from the stories told by nurses and patients. These stories define and explain caring as a virtue in nursing practice. According to both MacIntyre (1981) and Hauerwas (1974), humans are formed primarily by stories and metaphors, through which we learn to bring about variety in our existence. They entice us to discover the reality that should be, but which will not be until we act as if it is. The moral significance of principles and rules is contained in stories that give expression to the commitments we make if we desire to live our lives in a morally appropriate way.

Lives are not simply defined by our separate responses to particular situations; virtue embraces more than the single act. Virtue is like a theme in our lives through which the acts we do, or do not do, can be observed. To act requires an intention to develop character and virtue. Our character develops from the sustained attention that we give to the world. Virtue is the orientation of a person's whole life, shaped and given content by the stories through which we have learned to form the story of our lives.

Just as our lives are not defined by our separate acts, so moral judgments and decisions are more than what is determined by an observer. Our judgments of others are based not only on their acts or their solutions to problems; something less tangible is contempated—their total vision of life. This vision is illustrated in the thought pattern displayed continually in responses and conversations, word choice, sense of humor, and celebration. An actor's report provides more than the observer's descrption, for the telling action is inseparable from thought. Reasons do not produce my actions, but are embodied in them. Thus, in my study (Knowlden 1985), it was an important part of the data collection that I videotaped the nurse in the act of caring for the patient, so that both the nurse and the patient could tell the researcher later what they saw in the videotape that represented caring. The stories told by the nurses and the patients demonstrate an attempt to give coherence to events. "The essential unity of the self and its acts is the key to a correct theory of morality" (Hauerwas 1974, p.85).

The stories we use to organize our life are inherited from our culture and our particular autobiographical account (Hauerwas 1974). Caring is a cultural expectation that is held concerning nurses and is a basic philosophic premise of nursing. Florence Nightingale ([1869] 1970) noted the environment of caring in nursing in determining the outcome of a disease. Madeleine Leininger (1977) holds that caring is the essence of nursing. The stories told by nurses and patients reflect the caring that people have learned to expect from nurses.

In order to comprehend the logical development of a concept as a virtue, in this instance caring, three stages have to be identified. The first stage is the presence of a practice; the second is a narrative account of a single human life; while the third is an account of a moral tradition (MacIntyre 1981, 174).

An example of virtue in the first stage of a practice is revealed in a statement by a mother of twins: "[The nurse's] teaching is making sure that I'm not rushing the twins in their growing" (Knowlden 1985, 85). From a nursing perspective, the virtue implicit in this statement's meaning can be understood in isolation from its context. Placed in the narrative context of a human life, which is the second stage, the virtuous nature of the nurse's teaching becomes profound. The unwed mother of premature and developmentally delayed nine-month-old twins and their visiting nurse have known each other since the babies were discharged from the hospital. During videotape playback, the nurse talked about her nursing care with this mother.

I assisted her to get a home health aide because in the beginning she was so unsure with them; they were so premature. I have been able to find funding through Medicaide assistance and welfare assistance. There is also a project whose goal is to prevent child abuse with this type of child. Now I am preparing her for termination with the aide in the near future. We've also been investigating the need for day care, so she can return to work. . . . We've been talking about the possible responses of day-care workers to developmentally retarded twins. . . . Besides teaching her about the normal baby's development and her babies, I'm also teaching her about her own growth and development as a mother and as a person. I'm giving her emotional support; I'm reassuring her that life will go on, the children will grow up, and this is why we're planning. I let her know she's doing a good job. . . . Touching and playing with the babies, reviewing the schedule with her assists her to maintain a schedule with two individual babies. Everything was caring, visiting her, being supportive to her. Earlier in the relationship, there was more concrete teaching: this is the way you bathe, dress, etc. This physical stuff has been accomplished. Now there is a need for a new direction in growth and development, both hers and the babies' (Knowlden, 1985, raw data).

From the above account, certain factors become clear. First, the holistic nature of caring is demonstrated. Health teaching, planning for the future, and patient advocacy are provided in a relationship that expresses concern, emotional support, reassurance, and sustenance. Virtue here embraces more than the single act.

Second, it is clear that in this situation virtue has the meaning of a morally good action. But an action is not a virtue unless it is connected with an accompanying internal perspective. Virtue here means being a certain kind of person who judges and decides in a certain way. The nurse reveals her virtue when she states, "Now there is a need for a new direction in growth and development, both hers and the babies'." The behavior we observe is a clue to the presence of virtues in others. You cannot isolate motive from intention if the actor's meaning to be taken as an important part of moral activity. Intentionality cannot be reduced to the psycho-causal account of motivation (Gaffney 1979; Hauerwas 1974).

This nurse-patient situation also reveals that "there is no present which is not informed by an image of a future, an image which always presents itself in the form of a purpose—or a variety of ends or goals—towards which we are moving or failing to move in the present" (MacIntyre 1981, 200). The nurse and the patient together explore a vision of this young mother's future: what she needs, what she would like to do, and how the nurse and she can go about making it happen. Thus, hope for a happier future exists within the seeds of the present, and change and persistence coexist as part of our lives.

Also in this situation, virtue is revealed in the nurse's practice as more than just a set of technical skills. "What is distinctive of a practice is in part the way in which conceptions of the relevant goods and ends which the technical skills serve . . . are transformed and enriched by these extensions of human powers and by that regard for its own internal goods which is partially definitive of each particular or type of practice" (MacIntyre 1981, 180).

MacIntyre also indicates that to be in a practice is to enter into an alliance not only with contemporary practice, but also with others whose practices have preceded you. This is the third stage of the development of virtue.

To enter into a practice is to accept the authority of standards of excellence, obedience to rules, the achievement of goods, and the inadequacy of one's own performance as judged by them. It means that one must subject one's own attitudes, choices, preferences, and tastes to the practice. Generally in the realm of practices, the authority of standards acts to rule out all subjective and emotive analyses of judgment (MacIntyre 1981, 177).

However, in this analysis of virtue and caring, the emotional and subjective aspects are included as a necessary part of the whole.

In the following example, in order to demonstrate this third stage of the development of caring as a virtue, the nurse purposely used the videotape playback to gain greater knowledge about her practice. "An adequate sense of tradition manifests itself in its grasp of future possibilities which the past makes available to the present" (MacIntyre 1981, 207). The patient is a fifty-seven-year-old widow with a diabetic ulcer on her left foot. The nurse has found this patient challenging. In a sense, the challenge itself is interesting, for it can be considered a virtue "to have an adequate sense of the traditions to which one belongs or which confront one" (MacIntyre, 1981, 207). "As I listen, I sense the change in my voice at the difficulty I experience with this patient. I'm not looking at her. . . . I'm demonstrating caring concern via interest in the foot, touching, hands on . . . while hearing and responding. . . . I conclude that I show adequate concern in rendering care. I focus on the patient holistically" (Knowlden 1985, raw data).

Stories about nursing can be presented as part of the theory of caring in nursing as virtue, and thus can be central to educating us into the virtues. "We become, through our history, tellers of stories that aspire to truth" (MacIntyre 1981, 201). In the above nurse-patient situations, the stories aspire to tell the truth about nurse caring. Principles without stories are subject to diverse interpretations. Stories, even without the delineation of principles, have a way of distinctly indicating the actions and the practices that reveal the virtue expressed by the story.

The development of the fully human person includes the development of virtue. Virtue involves a free choice of positive values, especially those related to other humans. The development of virtue is essentially related to the human community. It is fundamental to our lives together that all human beings be considered morally deserving of just treatment, regardless of their merits, culture, or position. In that sense, all human beings constitute a basic moral community, but not a univocal community.

Moreover, a moral community compels the specific attitudes and actions that are virtues to be directed toward other persons in response to a particular sphere of values. Moral language does not just describe what is; it describes how we ought to see and direct our world (Crossin 1985). A broad understanding of people, language, and communication assists us in comprehending other human beings. For the nurse, understanding people, language, and communication facilitates a therapeutic nurse patient relationship. In my study, the nurses gained information about their practice by viewing the videotape. This enabled them to comprehend the caring in their practice, to learn about themselves and their patients, to perceive therapeutic nurse-patient relationships, to understand how their practice fitted into the traditional moral expectation that nursing is caring, and to grasp how their communication was therapeutic. Communication theorists postulate that the two aspects to communication are content (knowledge of the world) and relationship, and that content and relationship are integral and complementary in every communication (Watzlawick et al. 1967). Understanding the communication process enables the nurse to experience the successful results of nursing and the patient to experience health. The communication of a nurse-patient relationship that is therapeutic constitutes the essential caring in nursing. The therapeutic nurse-patient relationship is the tool through which caring in nursing becomes a virtue.

As Pehnix (1964) indicated, the distinctive goal of human existence is the realization of meaning. Meaning consists of the ability to:

(a) communicate intelligibly and forcefully,
(b) organize the experience of sense into significant generalizations and theories with predictive power,
(c) express the inner life in moving aesthetic constructions,
(d) relate to others and to oneself with acceptance and love,
(e) act with deliberate responsibility, and
(f) coordinate meanings into an integrated vision and commitment (Phenix 1964, 232).

The nurses and the patients who participated in my 1985 study were able to realize this goal—the meaning of nurse caring—through viewing the videotape of the nurse-patient situation. Meaning was made evident through the stories that the videotape presented and through the stories the nurses and patients told about their experience together. Virtues manifest and promote wholeness to the extent that they are rooted in the activation of a deep knowledge of the self and of the basic freedom by which persons commit themselves. Caring in nursing is a holistic construct made apparent in nursing practice as a virtue through nurses' actions and attitudes, which are reflected by the deep knowledge they have of themselves as committed caregivers.

# References

Beauchamp, T. and J. Childress. 1983. *Principles of biomedical ethics*, 2d ed. New York: Oxford University Press.

Carper, Barbara. 1979. The ethics of caring. In *Advances in Nursing Science* 1 (3):11–19.

Crossin, John W. 1985. *What Are They Saying About Virtue?* Mahwah, NJ: Paulist Press.

Erikson, Erik H. 1964. *Insight & Responsibility.* New York: W. W. Norton.

Gaffney, James. 1979. *Newness of Life.* Ramsey, NJ: Paulist Press.

Hauerwas, Stanley. 1974. The self as story: A reconsideration of the relation of religion and morality from the agent's perspective. In *Vision and Virtue.* Notre Dame, IN: Fides.

Knowlden, Virginia. 1985. *The Meaning of Caring in the Nursing Role.* Ann Arbor, MI: University Microfilms #8525485.

Leininger, M. 1977. Caring: The essence and central focus of nursing. *American Nurses' Foundation, Nursing Research Reports* 12(1):2–14.

MacIntyre, Alasdair. 1981. *After Virtue.* Notre Dame, IN: University of Notre Dame Press.

Mayeroff, Milton. 1971. *On Caring.* New York: Harper & Row.

Nightingale, Florence. (1869) 1970. *Notes on Nursing.* Princeton: Vertex book.

Phenix, Philip H. 1964. *Realms of Meaning.* New York: McGraw-Hill.

Watzlawick, P., J.H. Beavin, and D.D. Jackson. 1967. *Pragmatics of Human Communication.* New York: W.W. Norton.

*Webster's New Collegiate Dictionary.* 1974. Springfield, MA: G. C. Merriam.

# Oral Expression and Perceptions of Care with Ethical Implications

*Pamela Stinson Kidd, R.N., M.S.N., Ph.D., C.E.N.*

9

Caring can only be demonstrated and practiced effectively interpersonally. This study was designed to elicit how emergency nurses viewed caring through language use. A descriptive survey approach was used to address several research questions: What are the linguistic norms for the term *caring* used by nurses who work in emergency settings? Is there a relationship between the degree of transitivity, nominalization, and impersonalization used with the word *caring* and certain demographic characteristics of the emergency nurse? What are emergency nurses' perceptions of caring behaviors? Twenty-five conveniently sampled emergency nurses participated in an open-ended interview. The data were analyzed qualitatively and quantitatively. No one was informed that speech was a unit of analysis. Correlations between demographic variables and oral expression of caring were not statistically significant. Exploratory data analysis suggested that emergency nurses with less educational preparation and less than ten years of emergency nursing experience used caring in a personal, active, and action-focused manner. Caring was most often used in a low transitive form with a high use of nominalization and a high degree of impersonalization, which means that, linguistically, caring was being used impersonally, formally, and without involvement. Emergency nurses identified certain behaviors as caring in nature, which involved personalization, action, and participation. The linguistic choices used in the study may not be an effective strategy for meeting the goals of caring.

The purpose of this paper is to analyze language patterning of emergency nurses when they use the word *caring*. Norms among emergency nurses are presented, followed by a discussion of how linguistic norms relate to the ethical responsibility of emergency nurses as regards caring.

Nursing, as a profession, is based on the moral code of obligation, which is personified in the concept of service and respect for human life (Carper 1978). When viewed linguistically, caring can provide insight as an ethical response into the moral behavior of nurses. Caring requires a philosophy of commitment toward respecting and preserving humanity, and can only be effectively demonstrated and practiced interpersonally (Watson 1985). When nurses depersonalize discourse, the patient and nurse are not participating in a mutual interchange, and this diminishes effective caring. Morality requires two feelings: sentiment of natural caring and memories of caring and being cared for (Noddings 1984). Gilligan (1982), whose views on the development of morality focus on the notions of responsibility and care, has stressed the importance of dialogue, since it allows each individual to be understood in his or her own terms. The manner in which caring is expressed becomes as important as the pure description of the caring experience (Watson 1985). Care phenomena can be discovered by examining language, since social structure and worldview influence care through language and the environment (Leininger 1985). Thus, examination of how caring is orally expressed by emergency nurses can provide information on the influence of the social structure on the emergency nursing caring process as the foundation of ethical response. The commitment to caring has been viewed as an ethical ideal (Noddings 1984).

## Literature Review

Speech can be viewed as an act of identity since it provides a structure a person can use in locating the self or person in the world. A person can identify several social groups by language use. Lepage states behavior can be modified in order to match a group's use of language if the person is able to: (a) identify the group, (b) observe and analyze the group's behavior, (c) be internally motivated to adapt behavior accordingly, and (d) verbally adapt one's language use (cited in Hudson 1983, 27). An assumption in this study was that emergency nurses would use caring based on a group norm. This was derived from the belief that emergency nurses see themselves as a group because of their defined specialty of practice. Information about the group norm, and determining whether a modification in the norm occurs, could provide insights into a change in the linguistic use of caring. Caring may be expressed differently according to the length of time spent in the emergency setting.

The influence of social network on linguistic variables, as conveyed demographically, has been addressed. Trudgill (1975) explored the relationship between geographic location and the use of language. The influence of race, occupation, kinship, socio-economic status, and religion on the use of lexical items and pronunciation has also been explored (Labov 1972). There is no agreement in the literature on which social factors provide the best predictor of linguistic use since so much variation exists between groups, yet it appears that different factors are relevant to different variables (Hudson 1983). This study attempted to identify which demographic factors of emergency nurses are significantly related to the linguistic use of caring.

The role of language in nursing has not been extensively studied. The only available study addressed perception change of unsociable behavior through language restructuring (Neizo and Lanza 1984). An implication of that study was that mental health nurses could assist a patient in altering his or her language style in order to change dysfunctional perceptions associated with violence. The study explored deletion, nominalization, and impersonalization as language violations. Some of these same violations were explored in this study on emergency nurses' linguistic use of caring.

Shuy has explored the mystique of technical vocabulary (cited in Mehan 1983). Technical language can be used as a way of indicating superiority, advanced education, and the possession of specialized knowledge. When technical language is used, the grounds for negotiating meaning are removed (Mehan 1983). When speakers and hearers do not share the same language, the hearers do not have the expertise to challenge what is said. If nurses use technical language when discussing caring, it is reasonable to assume that patients, who do not share that language, cannot question the legitimacy of the behaviors associated with it.

To summarize, little is known about the linguistic use of caring in nursing. Caring does not have a single meaning in all nursing contexts.

## Conceptual Orientation

The word *caring* is derived from the old English and Gothic words *carian, kara,* or *Karon* (Gaut 1983). As a noun, *care* was related to *grief* or *bed of sickness.* Earlier indications of caring included: *to attend, to regard,* and *to protect.* In scholarly writings, the notion of care had several referents, such as love, concern, and understanding (Gaut 1983).

Several linguists have identified characteristics of discourse that can be evaluated. Those that address involvement, completion, action, and personalization were used in the study, based on the assumption that caring refers to love, concern, and understanding, and thus requires these properties.

Transitivity refers to the effectiveness of transferring action and is a property of verbs and verb clauses (Hopper and Thompson 1980). Clauses with high transitivity are action oriented, involving the transfer of a completed action from one participant to another (Hopper and Thompson 1980). There are a total of ten components to transitivity. The three major components—kinesis, aspect, and number of participants—are used in this study. Each of the components can be ranked on a continuum and then added to produce a transitivity score (Hopper and Thompson 1980). Kinesis refers to the actual transferring of action from one participant to another (as in "Bob is caring for the patient"). Aspect refers to the completion of an action. The statement "I introduced myself to the patient as a way of showing caring" includes a completed action and thus aspect is present. Whenever two or more participants are included in the discourse, it is considered a highly transitive discourse. An example of a highly transitive statement that includes kinesis, aspect, and two participants, is: "The role of the emergency nurse is caring for the patient until he or she is able to take care of him- or herself."

Nominalization is a characteristic of backgrounding, which provides extra information that is not central to the proposition. Nominalizations are generally very low in transitivity and are formal and less personal (Ohashi 1978). They usually have one participant. An example of a nominalization is: "You are under no legal obligation to fulfill an incorrect physician order"; versus the denominalized form: "You are not obliged to fulfill an incorrect physician order." The nominalized sentence is less dynamic, more formal, and less personal.

Personalization involves the use of personal pronouns, resulting in an informal utterance (Ohashi, 1978). A person who speaks in generalizations and does not address any particular individual or group is depersonalizing (Neizo and Lanza 1984). A depersonalization statement would be: "Explaining procedures is good for decreasing anxiety." A personalized form would be: "Explaining procedures will decrease a patient's anxiety."

A total linguistic score was derived for each informant by adding the degree of transitivity, nominalization, and personalization together for each use of the word *caring*. A documented relationship is present between these three properties. "Nominalizations are extremely low in transitivity: since by themselves they never make assertions and tend to have only one participant which is furthermore typically impersonal" (Hopper & Thompson 1980, 252).

## Introduction to the Study

This study was designed to elicit how emergency nurses viewed caring through language use. There were two goals: (a) the identification of linguistic norms for the oral expression of care, and (b) a comparison of the linguistic norms of the group with caring behaviors identified within the same group. The researcher speculated that nurses who used detached, depersonalized discourse in discussing caring would have longer tenures of working in emergency settings and would demonstrate impersonalization as a coping behavior. Since there was no previous research addressing the linguistic expression of caring in this population, an exploratory design was selected.

## Research Method

The study used a descriptive survey approach, which is appropriate for a topic that has not been researched in-depth (Wilson 1985). Several research questions were addressed: What are the linguistic norms for the term *caring* used by nurses who work in emergency settings? Is there a relationship between the degree of transitivity, nominalization, and impersonalization used with the word *caring* and certain demographic characteristics of the emergency nurse? What are emergency nurses' perceptions of caring behaviors?

An open-ended interview guide was used as the method to collect data. Data were transcribed and coded by the researcher, then analyzed qualitatively, using a format identified by Spradley (1979). Relationships were explored using descriptive statistics and exploratory data analysis (Hartwig and Dearing 1979).

### Sample

Twenty-five conveniently selected emergency nurses participated in one thirty- to forty-five-minute tape-recorded interview. Tandem informants were used in lieu of repeated interviews with the same informant (Spradley 1979). A conscious effort was made to collect information from emergency nurses who worked in a variety of settings within the United States.

Different levels of educational preparations and of work experience in the emergency setting existed within the sample group. Diversity in the sample provided greater credibility to the assumption that emergency nurses, regardless of extraneous factors, share linguistic norms for the oral expression of caring. All informants signed an informed consent and each informant was told that he or she was participating in a study exploring emergency nurses perception of caring. No one was informed that speech was a unit of analysis, thereby assuring that informants would not place undue concentration on the semantic or grammatical quality of their responses.

## Recording of Responses: Oral Expression of Care

Each time the informant used the word *caring* in the interview, a total linguistic score (TLS) was calculated by the researcher based on the degree of transitivity, nominalization, and personalization present. A transitivity score was calcuated for each informant, which consisted of the three components—participants, kinesis, and aspect. Two or more participants were scored as 20 points. One participant was scored as 10 points. The presence of action (kinesis) was scored 20 points, while the absence of action was scored 10 points. Aspect was coded as either completed action (20 points) or incomplete (10 points). Thus, the range of transitivity scores possible for each use of caring was 30 to 60 points. The presence of nominalization was scored as 10 points, its absence was 20 points. Personalization resulted in a score of 20 points, while impersonalization was scored as 10 points. A total linguistic score of 100 points was possible for each oral use of caring. A total linguistic score of 100 points indicated a personalized, informal, active use of caring. The total mean linguistic score for each interview was derived by adding the TLS for each use of caring and dividing by the number of times caring was used.

The data were analyzed for frequency and percentage values by SPSS-PC programs (SPSS 1986). Correlations for interval variables were obtained by using Pearson correlation coefficients. The relationships between demographic variables and scores were analyzed by the use of chi-square cross-tabulations and Fischer exact probabilities where the sample size was less than 20 cases in a $2 \times 2$ table (Hays 1981). A probability level of .05 was used in the study. The data were graphed and analyzed using Exploratory Data Analysis (EDA) in order to identify subtle trends that may appear statistically insignificant because of a small sample size (Hartwig and Dearing 1979). Exploratory data analysis uses visual displays (such as box plots and graphs) to examine relationships within the data.

## Recording of Responses: Perceptions of Caring

The interviews were initiated using a grand tour question: "Why are you in emergency nursing?" Later in the interview, comparative questions were posed, such as: "How is safeguarding different from being there as an example of caring?" Differences between identified behaviors were used to structure a taxonomy. Consistencies in the interviews suggested themes for caring behaviors. The final taxonomy and themes were reflective of emergency nurses' caring behaviors. One of the informants reviewed the final taxonomy and themes and confirmed the findings, which helped to enhance the credibility of the analysis.

## Findings

### Expression of Caring

Demographic data were available for twenty-three of the twenty-five informants. As can be seen in table 9.1, a broad representation was obtained in the sample. The "average" informant was female, with seven to twelve years of emergency nursing experience, and was a staff nurse employed in a private, non-profit hospital emergency department. Although ten states were represented, the majority of the

TABLE 9.1
Summary of Demographic Characteristics of the Subjects (N = 23)

| Variable | Number | Percent |
|---|---|---|
| *Years of ER experience* | | |
| 1–6 | 4 | 17. 4 |
| 7–14 | 12 | 52. 2 |
| 15 or more | 7 | 30. 4 |
| *Educational level* | | |
| ADN | 5 | 21. 7 |
| Diploma | 5 | 21. 7 |
| BSN | 5 | 21. 7 |
| MSN or PhD | 8 | 34. 8 |
| *Position in emergency nursing* | | |
| Staff Nurse | 11 | 47. 8 |
| Educator (CE or Academia) | 4 | 17. 4 |
| Administrator | 5 | 27. 1 |
| Trauma Nurse Coordinator | 3 | 13. 0 |
| *Type of institution* | | |
| Public | 10 | 43. 5 |
| Private | 13 | 56. 5 |
| Non-Profit | 17 | 73. 9 |
| Profit | 6 | 26. 1 |
| *Sex* | | |
| Female | 20 | 87. 0 |
| Male | 3 | 13. 0 |
| *Location* | | |
| Arizona | 1 | 4. 3 |
| California | 3 | 13. 0 |
| Kentucky | 3 | 13. 0 |
| Michigan | 1 | 4. 3 |
| New Mexico | 1 | 4. 3 |
| New York | 2 | 8. 7 |
| Ohio | 2 | 8. 7 |
| Oklahoma | 2 | 8. 7 |
| Pennsylvania | 3 | 13. 0 |
| Texas | 5 | 21. 7 |

informants were from Texas. These facts are typical of the emergency nursing population as a whole except for the educational level and geographic location of the nurse. The majority of emergency nurses are usually associate degree or diploma prepared (personal communication, ENA, 1988); here BSN, MSN or Ph.D.

Total linguistic scores did not vary markedly. The mean score was 61.64 with a range from 50 to 98. Only one informant had a total linguistic score that was reflective of a highly personalized and active use of caring (see table 9.2).

Descriptive statistics did not reveal significant relationships between demographic characteristics and linguistic scores. Exploratory data analysis revealed

TABLE 9.2

Total Linguistic Score for Informants

| | Score | Frequency | Percent |
|---|---|---|---|
| Total Linguistic Score | 50 | 4 | 16 |
| (transitivity + nominalization + impersonalization) | | | |
| | 53 | 4 | 16 |
| | 54 | 1 | 4 |
| | 55 | 1 | 4 |
| | 57 | 1 | 4 |
| | 58 | 1 | 4 |
| | 60 | 2 | 8 |
| | 61 | 1 | 4 |
| | 65 | 3 | 12 |
| | 68 | 2 | 8 |
| | 72 | 1 | 4 |
| | 73 | 1 | 4 |
| | 75 | 2 | 8 |
| | 98 | 1 | 4 |

that emergency nurses with less educational preparation scored higher, which could be interpreted as an oral use of caring in a personal, active, and action-completed manner. Emergency nurses with less than ten years of emergency nursing experience used caring in a similar pattern. However, these patterns were not strong enough to produce a significant correlation with the chi-square statistic.

## Perception of Caring

The category "activities that demonstrate caring" was identified and was subdivided into helping, supporting, and coping activities. Differences between the subcategories were based on the presence of communication behaviors, preparation behaviors, advocacy behaviors, and the impact of the activity on the physiologic status of the patient. Two themes consistently surfaced in the interviews: (a) communication is a primary vehicle for most caring activities, and (b) caring is a global term for all activities of the emergency nurse (See table 9.3).

## Discussion

A norm for the oral expression of caring exists for nurses in emergency settings. Caring is most often used in a low transitive form with a high use of nominalization and a high degree of impersonalization, which means that, linguistically, caring is being used impersonally, formally, and without involvement. The linguistic norm was consistent across the sample as evidenced by non-significant correlations between the demographic variables and the total linguistic scores. However, when the data was graphed visually, exploratory data analysis revealed an emerging pattern of oral expression. Nurses who have more education and a long tenure of experience in emergency nursing use caring more universally, but in a less participative sense. Re-examiniation with a larger sample size may confirm the existence of this pattern.

TABLE 9.3

Perception of Caring Behaviors

| | | | |
|---|---|---|---|
| **Helping** | preparation | expedite existing patient care<br>check out equipment<br>get support services<br>go through worst-case scenario<br>get supplies | |
| | when patient arrives | find out circumstances of event<br>start IV<br>take care of physiologic needs<br>draw blood<br>set up trays<br>open crash cart & give meds<br>get the doctor | |
| **Supporting** | | check on patient frequently | |
| | | reinforce information | encourage patient to ask questions<br>get to point |
| | | explain<br>get family | say family is on its way |
| | | try to get other people in ER<br>say "I am here for you"<br>say "There is somebody with you"<br>follow up | |
| | | inform | identify self as caregiver<br>tell them your name |
| | take care of needs | verbalize for patient<br>acknowledge his/her hurt<br>call patient by name | |
| | communication by nurse | talk into patient's ear<br>maintain eye contact<br>let patient see your emotions | |
| **Assisting with coping** | give patient a sense of control | give patient choices<br>clarify what the nurse is doing<br>illustrate what is going to happen<br>bring patient up to the present<br>orient patient<br>get permission | |
| | comfort measures | touch<br>talk<br>provide privacy<br>take time to be with patient | |
| | empathy | control my anxiety<br>be honest<br>say "We know that accidents happen when you are least prepared" | |

To the emergency nurse, *caring* was a complex term. The informants described it as involving three major concepts: helping, coping, or supporting activities. Compared with existing research in this area, the informants considered caring behaviors, which mainly addressed the patient's physiological needs and technical competence, such as drawing blood or giving medications, important to the subcategory of helping (Larson 1984; L. Brown 1981; Ford 1981; Henry 1975). The relationships between helping, supporting, and assisting with coping were identified and explained by informants, along with the relationship of these three to caring expressions. Data from this study supported the three concepts of helping, supporting, and assisting with coping as demonstrated by the following examples.

Helping was seen as a more task-oriented and interdependent action. As one informant stated, "Helping is taking someone from point *A* in hopes of reaching point *B*, some sort of progression in their medical care, their physiological changes." Another informant stated, "Helping is interdependent. It's assisting or doing something, hands-on tasks."

The data revealed that supporting had a non-physical focus and was viewed as an "all-nursing" function. The informants' interview texts reveal these characteristic statements about support: "Support is more on the psychosocial realm than physical. I'm not thinking of it as a way of talking in terms of supporting a limb that needs traction." "I certainly would not need anybody else to tell my how to support someone, like a physician's order. It's definitely initiated by myself."

Assisting with coping, as supported by the data, involved the patient as an active participant. For example, one informant stated: "They start to deal with it and you step in and help them sort things out."

Emergency nurses spoke of caring in a more general nature, a foundation on which their practice was based. They stated: "Caring guides me to do what turns out to be supportive," and "Caring is your baseline of where you're coming from."

## Ethical Implications

Social networks provide goals and desires that motivate the actions of individuals. For example, if an individual's family supports a strong work ethic in order to purchase goods, the chances are greater that the individual will be motivated to work and purchase. Certain cummulative strategies serve as means to achieve these goals, and these strategies suggest certain linguistic choices (P. Brown, 1979). Emergency nurses make linguistic choices that are influenced by the goals they wish to achieve. In sum, findings from this investigation showed that emergency nurses did identify certain behaviors as caring in nature—behaviors involving personalization, action, and participation, such as being honest, acknowledging the patient's hurt, and saying, "I am here for you." However, the discourse they used when discussing caring itself was depersonalized and formal.

The linguistic choices used in this study may not be an effective strategy for meeting the goals of caring and determining an ethical response. The caring one must address the one-cared-for with an attitude of receptivity, otherwise the one-cared-for will feel like an object (Noddings 1984). Noddings also states that "words and acts of caring must confirm that the one caring does care or the message is ambiguous and the recipient will either feel uncared for or that it's permissible to hurt those we care for" (1984, 120). Patients may be interpreting emergency nurses' oral expression of caring, its linguistic use, as impersonal, passive, and formal and may feel that their relationship with the nurse is uncaring in nature. Although emergency nurses perceive caring as an interpersonal event that actively involves the patient, as indicated by the subcategory of coping activities, perception is not enough. Speech acts are intrisically potent because they presuppose various things about the addressee (P. Brown 1979). By using the word *caring* in an intransitive form, the emergency nurse is treating the patient linguistically as backgrounded, impersonal material. Receptivity appears essential to caring and is conveyed with Noddings's general perspective in that the cared-for experiences differences when being cared for, and being cared for enhances or diminishes attitudes conveyed to the person being cared for (Noddings, 1984, 60–61). If patients are interpreting the oral expression of caring used in this study, human caring is absent, and thus the foundation of ethical response is absent also.

By becoming aware of how nurses verbally express caring and the relationship of the verbal use to the ethical values being expressed, the possibility exists for language to be modified in a manner that promotes "a feeling of being cared for," and that is ethically congruent with emergency nurses' perceptions of the caring process. Otherwise, the possibility exists that emergency nurses may come to view caring passively and to look at patients as "backgrounded" components of an impersonal process.

## References

Brown, L. 1981. Behaviors of nurses perceived by hospitalized patients as indicators of care. Ph.D. diss. University of Colorado at Boulder. *Dissertation Abstracts International* 43, 4361B.

Brown, P. 1979. How and why are women more polite: Some evidence from a Mayan community. In *Women and language in literature and society*, edited by S. McConnels-Guet, R. Borker, P. Furman, 111–134. New York: Praeger.

Carper, B. 1978. Fundamental patterns of knowing in nursing. *Advances in Nursing Science* 1(1): 13–23.

Ford, M. (1981). Nurse professionals and the caring process. Ph.D. diss., University of Northern Colorado. *Dissertation Abstracts International* 43, 967B–968B.

Gaut, D. 1983. Development of a theoretically adequate description of caring. *Western Journal of Nursing Research* 5(4): 313–23.

Gilligan, C. 1982. *In a different voice: Psychological theory and women's development.* Cambridge: Harvard University Press.

Hartwig, F., and B. Dearing. 1979. Exploratory data analysis. In *Quantitative applications in the social sciences, Series No. 07-0716, edited by J. Sullivan and R. Niemi, Beverly Hills: Sage Publications.*

Hays, W. 1981. *Statistics*, 3rd ed. New York: Holt, Rinehart & Winston.

Henry, O. 1975. Nurse behaviors perceived by patients as indicators of caring. Ph.D. diss., Catholic University *Dissertation Abstracts International* 36, 2652B.

Hopper, P., and S. Thompson. 1980. Transitivity in grammar and discourse. *Language: Journal of the Linguistic Society of America* 56(20): 251–95.

Hudson, R. 1983. *Sociolinguistics.* Oxford: Cambridge University Press.

Labov, W. 1972. *Language in the inner city.* Philadelphia: University of Pennsylvania Press.

Larson, P. 1984. Oncology patients and professional nurses important nurse caring behaviors. Ph.D. diss., University of California, San Francisco.

Leininger, M. 1985. Transcultural care diversity and universality: A theory of nursing. *Nursing and health care* 6(4): 209–12.

Mehan, H. 1983. The role of language and the language of role in institutional decision making. *Language in Society* 12(1): 187–211.

Neizo, B., and M. Lanza. 1984. Post violence dialogue: Perception of change through language restructuring. *Issues in Mental Health Nursing* 6: 150–56.

Noddings, N. 1984. *Caring: A feminine approach to ethics and moral education.* Berkeley: University of California Press.

Ohashi, Y. 1978. *English style, grammatical and semantic approach.* Rowley, MA: Newbury House.

Spradley, J. 1979. *The ethnographic interview.* New York: Holt, Rinehart & Winston.

SPSS Incorporated. 1986. *SPSS/PC users guide,* 2d ed. Chicago, Author.

Trudgill, P. 1975. Linguistic change and diffusion: Description and explanation in sociolinguistic dialect geography. *Language in Society* 2: 215–46.

Watson, J. 1985. *Nursing: Human science and human care. A theory of nursing.* Norwalk, CT: Appleton-Century-Crofts.

Wilson, H. 1985. *Research in nursing.* Menlo Park, CA: Addison-Wesley.

# Development of the Need for Tenderness as a Theoretical Model for Caring: Application to Nursing Education

*Marilyn Miller, R.N., M.A., and Laura C. Zamora, R.N., M.A.*

**10**

In order to promote the caring critical to ethical action in nursing, the dynamics of caring require clarification. Useful to this clarification is the concept of tenderness, which was central to interpersonal theorists' explanation of human emotional growth. Tenderness-need theory is elaborated as the sequential, interpersonal development of both the need and capacity for tenderness. The relation of tenderness-need development to caring behaviors is described. Applications are made to promotion of caring in developing a nursing curriculum. Particular emphasis is placed on teacher-student interaction, with attention to the distinction between power and tenderness orientations in relationships. Research implications are discussed.

A philosophical commitment to caring as a standard of conduct makes this an ethic central to nursing practice, education, and research. Despite this commitment to caring and the proliferation of interest in nursing ethics during the past ten years, the application of such ethical principles as autonomy, beneficence, and justice to the human condition is often unclear.

Ethicists have noted the connection between interpersonal theory and ethics. Specifically, they have observed that interpersonal relationships are at the heart of ethical questions in nursing, and that morality and ethics are social in their origins (Davis and Aroskar 1983; Curtin and Flaherty 1982). Interpersonal theory, as formulated by Sullivan (1953), used a developmental approach. Sullivan explained how, from birth onward, "a very capable animal becomes a person" and how this transformation is brought about through the influence of other people, solely for the purpose of living with other people in some sort of social organization (Sullivan 1953, 5). Sullivan and other interpersonal theorists (Pearce and Newton 1963) described how emotional growth proceeds in steps from total dependence of the infant to a mature adult's total independence from the original matrix—the family of origin. The human need for tenderness was inferred by Sullivan as central to interpersonal development. The interpersonal development of the need for tenderness was elaborated and expanded by Pearce and Newton. In this paper, the need for tenderness is defined as those generic human tensions (such as the needs for food, air, contact, warmth), the relief of which requires cooperation by another (Sullivan 1953, 40). The tenderness response is defined as a "response to the other's true needs for growth, with a degree of accuracy appropriate to the urgency of the need at the particular moment of development" (Pearce and Newton 1963, 170). Together, the need for tenderness and the capacity to respond tenderly define tenderness. The sequential, interpersonal development of the need and capacity for tenderness throughout life, as presented by Sullivan and Pearce and Newton, is called by the authors "tenderness-need theory."

The purposes of this paper are: (1) to discuss how tenderness-need theory explains the development of human caring behaviors, (2) to describe how problems in caring can arise from an inadequate understanding or distorted development of the need for human tenderness, and (3) to offer suggestions for the use of tenderness-need theory in nursing education as a means of strengthening the ethic of caring in nursing practice. While a full discussion of tenderness-need theory will not be presented, major concepts that constitute the theory will be described to show the relationship of tenderness to human caring.

## Tenderness-Need Theory

Tenderness is developed interpersonally through the process of validation. Validation refers to the confirmation by one person of another's experience, the process of one person experiencing satisfaction in the other's individuation (Pearce and Newton 1963, 31). As a result, the other person integrates the experience consciously and productively. For example, to the extent that parents take pleasure in an infant's needs for food, warmth, or touch, that infant will experience these generic tensions as needs in consciousness and will develop his or her own capacities for satisfaction of those needs. An infant's needs to which parents react with indifference, a negative mood, or a forbidding gesture, will continue unsatisfied, and will tend to be repressed from the infant's consciousness. The tender quality of these early interactions is critical because they initiate the capacity for tenderness in the infant (Pearce and Newton 1963, 15).

To the extent that parental validation is conflicted or unavailable, developing children will require alternate validation of their needs by other adults. When parents provide such alternate validation, they respond accurately to the needs of the child and thereby promote the expansion of his or her capacity for tenderness. Opposition by parents to other adults having an important influence on the child is often rationalized as being for the child's protection or own good. But this opposition usually serves the parents' goal of long-range control over the child, with the result of entrenching the child's dependence on the parents' values.

Although adult validators continue to be important until the child reaches adulthood, validation by peers becomes progressively more essential. The degree to which an adult will be able to have tender relationships with peers depends on this progressive validation.

The validated capacities become the productive functions of an individual's personality. The productive functions include all those needs that the individual can satisfy if the means for satisfaction are available (Pearce and Newton 1963, 27). For example, major needs of infants include the provision for their physiology, perception, and movement needs and for their active and energetic needs relating to space and objects. To the degree that parents validate these needs, the infant's capacity for curiosity and pleasure begins to develop into productive functions.

For the purposes of this paper, the authors focus on the productive functions that are emerging and expanding during adolescence and young adulthood, since it is during these developmental periods that people commonly begin their study of nursing. Adolescents and young adults are still ignorant in many ways and may be financially dependent on parents. Nonetheless they are responsible at these stages of development for the progressive organization of their own growth, and should no longer be thought of as children. They require opportunities to develop a series of love and friendship relationships with individuals of both sexes and of varying backgrounds. In this way they can potentially find validation for any human capacity.

In addition to the productive functions, the conscious personality includes all those patternings of perception, thought, feeling, and action that serve to keep unsatisfied needs out of awareness. These are called security operations (Pearce and Newton 1963; Sullivan 1953). Security operations are experienced as protective in that they help to avoid anxiety that results in disorganization, disorientation, and difficulty in concentrating. However, security operations are essentially unproductive in that they interfere with an accurate view of what is going on.

Looking at adolescent and young-adult experience, one often finds that there is considerable conflict between the need for expanded relatedness with peers and the restrictive psychological dependence on parents. To protect themselves emotionally, young people may, for example, seek new friends, but within the framework of parental prejudices. Thus their capacity for tenderness—and caring—continues to be somewhat restricted.

The particular productive function the authors are addressing is the capacity to make caring choices—that is, to exercise and expand the need for tenderness in self and others. The contexts the authors are specifically considering are health care and education, where ideas may be unfamiliar, directives unclear, and prohibitions many and conflicting. Tenderness-need theory postulates that one's ability to be tender, that is, to respond accurately to the needs of others, depends on one's experience in having one's own needs validated by significant others (Pearce and Newton 1963, 170). To the extent that people understand the limitations of those experiences and act on that understanding, their choices will be rooted in a capacity for tenderness rather than in security operations. To that extent behavior will incorporate the ethic of caring.

## Tenderness-Need Theory Applied to Nursing Education

"Caring is the central and unifying domain for the body of knowledge and practices in nursing" (Leininger 1981, 3). The philosophical and scientific bases that define and support caring as nursing's central focus continue to be extensively developed by nursing scholars (Leininger 1981 1984; Watson 1979). The contribution of tenderness-need theory to the work of these scholars is that the theory expands the knowledge base available for promotion of caring behaviors.

Using the development of the need and capacity for tenderness as the theoretical basis for caring, one can assume that most students come into nursing with some capacity for caring. That is, the students' experiences have been sufficiently validated for them to understand clearly some of their needs and to respond accurately to the needs of patients and peers. One can also assume that the capacity for tenderness may be underdeveloped and fragile, which will present the greatest obstacle to excellent nursing practice, including the clear thinking and emotional depth required for ethical decision making. Alternatively, one can view these deficits as the nurse educator's greatest challenge.

Of all the possible questions one might use to organize a curriculum in nursing, then, the central one is: How does one support the student's capacity for caring, free it and nurture it, within our society? In other words, using tenderness-need theory as a knowledge base for caring, how do we implement caring in the curriculum? A proposed model for the application of tenderness-need theory to a nursing curriculum includes three major components: program objective, conceptual framework, and process.

The first component, which directs all others, is a clear statement of the central program objective: to promote effective caring. This objective would incorporate the goal of caring, which is expansion of human need satisfaction in health and illness throughout the life span.

The second component is the conceptual framework: the major ideas that direct the selection of content and experience essential in fulfilling the central program objective. Following through with the theoretical model of tenderness, the authors emphasize tenderness-need theory as primary in a curriculum focused on caring. Tenderness-need theory is compatible with a number of components of caring already identified by nurse scholars and thus is a useful choice as a primary theory. Those specific components of caring to which the authors refer are: universality (Leininger 1981); human-needs orientation (Watson 1979); scientific and humanistic integration (Watson 1979); inherent themes of growth and health (Ray 1988); and interpersonal nature (Watson 1981). In order to develop the capacity for caring, then, other needs are taught in the context of the development of the need for tenderness. In other words, such human needs as relatedness, air, nutrition, activity, and aesthetics can be understood as generic tensions. Developing an awareness of and the capacity to satisfy these needs requires the cooperation of others. Within each category of need are productive functions that push for expansion in health and illness throughout the lifespan. Understanding the need for relatedness, for example, might entail the study of communication, perceptual thought, and emotional and sexual functions. Similarly, productive functions can be identified for all human need areas. These productive functions, the circumstances and styles in which these needs manifest themselves in individuals and groups, are of concern to nursing. A study of these needs would constitute a major component of nursing content and clinical experience. A beginning course in the nursing major, for example, would include specific content in tenderness-need theory as well as other needs identified as generic tensions and their related productive functions. Clinically, students would learn how to assess the need satisfaction of essentially well people in their homes, schools, places of work, or recreation. The skills of interviewing and physical examination, taught in conjunction with needs content, would enhance the students' ability to promote patients' awareness of needs, capacities for need satisfaction, and expansion of productive functions. Nursing care would be defined as a tenderness response, in that care would be aimed at cooperating with patients to validate and, where possible, relieve the tension of the particular manifest need; the overall goal would be to expand the patients' productive functions. The students' capacities to be accurate in this process would evolve as students progress through the curriculum. In subsequent nursing courses, for example, students would be assisted in intervening with needs and productive functions when there is illness or a change in people's lives.

Contributing theories enrich students' abilities to reflect upon making appropriate actions in relation to human needs. For example, anthropological theory contributes to students' appreciation of the ways in which a given culture promotes or inhibits expansion of productive functions. It helps them understand and respond effectively to variations in human expression while keeping in mind the universal needs. Bio-physical theory assists students in understanding the complexity and evolution of interacting systems of the human body as well as how humans interact with their environments in both health and illness. Sociopolitical and psychological theories shed light on human behavior and its relationship to individuals and groups in society. This is important not only from the standpoint of respecting the needs of an individual patient, but of enabling critical analyses of, and consequently accurate responses to, the needs of society. The humanities expand students' awareness of the richness and variety of human experience. Study of language, literature, philosophy, religion, and the fine arts, for example, offers opportunities to expand one's thinking about humanness as a dynamic and evolving condition. New ideas and change can then be viewed as productive and exciting.

Through understanding research processes, students learn about the ways in which human needs can be investigated and thus be better understood. The authors include the nursing process here as a level of research—a way of thinking dynamically about human problems.

The third component of curriculum is the "how"—the process by which students will integrate the capacity for caring. Since tenderness is an underpinning of caring and is developed interpersonally, it follows that a major means of promoting effective caring will be interpersonal. Therefore the student-teacher relationship is critical to the application of tenderness-need theory to education in nursing.

In implementing the student-teacher relationship, one must inevitably be concerned with the degree to which society is preoccupied with power orientation in relationships. A power-oriented relationship, as opposed to a tenderness-oriented relationship, is hostile to the satisfaction of needs and therefore to learning and growth. Such a preoccupation is often manifested in adult problems with authority, in tyrannical leadership styles, or in disregard for human needs. As an important restrictive function of most cultures, preoccupation with power deserves attention. For example, Klein (1963) documented statements of self-imagery among a group of male adults from an Andean culture, and the data showed that "the most frequently listed single theme is the view that all human relationships are essentially power-oriented and therefore hostile" (Klein 1963, 116). This view of relationships as power-oriented contributed to the subjects' inability to pursue and enjoy satisfactions that were in fact available to them in their daily lives.

There are parallels in our society. For example, the authoritarian structure of our educational institutions contributes to a power orientation in relationships among people in those institutions. The restrictiveness may not appear to be so great as among the Andeans in Klein's research. However, the hierarchical system often determines relationships and behaviors based more on who has power over whom than on mutual respect or the satisfaction of the needs of teachers, students, and patients. The preoccupation with power is in turn fueled by the actively restrictive nature of individual security operations. For example, demands from the top may be rationalized as being for the good of everyone, when in reality a few people at the top benefit.

Therefore, to relate with students in a way that promotes caring, teachers must transcend not only the limitations of their own experience, but the restrictiveness of the society as well. That is, the task of teachers is to encourage learning and to deal with or overcome unnecessary political societal barriers.

There are, of course, contingencies with educational institutions over which teachers have limited immediate control or influence. However, if nurse educators are functioning with students interests in mind, they can choose to respond accurately to the urgency of the students' true needs for growth, and thus promote a foundation for caring. When one applies tenderness-need theory to the student-teacher relationship, one recognizes that:

1. Students and teachers are both adults, not parents and children.

2. The student-teacher relationship is expert-client, where the expertise (teaching) needed by the client (student) is primarily reflective and facilitative, not power-oriented.

3. Encounters are directed toward the students' perceiving some benefit: validation, clarification, increased motivation to learn and care, increased competence in some productive function, or pleasure. Teachers benefit similarly in that they expand their knowledge as well as take pleasure in the students' growth.

4. Where behaviors in students or teachers are motivated by avoidance of anxiety, there will be serious and inevitable conflict with learning. For instance, student behavior that teachers label "failing," "problematic," or "unsatisfactory" may be efforts by students to avoid disorganization, disorientation, and difficulty in concentrating. Anxiety in the teacher, on the other hand, is typically avoided by moving out of a peer orientation and into a power orientation.

5. The relationship offers students a different experience from ones that have militated against growth. That means, for example, helping the student to change conceptions of the self as limited, incompetent, hopeless, or bad, rather than confirming such self-conceptions.

6. Ethical dilemmas posed in education and health care may be perceived as positive in that they confront students and teachers with the possibility of alternate experience, the opportunity to re-examine thinking and a situation in which to test theoretical approaches.

## Research Implications

Finally, there is the question of how to research this theory and its application to education and practice. The authors have observed that teachers, students, and patients engage in operations that obscure their needs for growth and productivity. Students, for example, are often compliant with testing procedures that many doubt and which continue to be presented as "necessary" by those in power. Theoretically compliance continues because to challenge the people in power symbolizes a challenge to the parents' values—an event that is unthinkable. In order to promote greater awareness of such patterns and thereby expand the human capacity for tenderness, it is necessary to study the relationship of tenderness-need development and caring in more systematic ways in our society and in others. In addition to the previously cited investigation by Klein (1963), the research of Stern (1985) and his colleagues in the United States may provide guidance. In studying the infant's developing sense of self, Stern devised protocols that yielded rich qualitative data in the area of infant-adult interaction, suggesting particularly how infants' behaviors reflect their interpersonal experience. Such approaches, with relevant modifications, could be applied to the study of the need for tenderness and its relation to caring behaviors in student-teacher and nurse-patient dyads.

## Summary

Since caring is the essence of nursing, nurse educators need to teach caring. Tenderness-need theory provides a basis for understanding caring. It suggests the need for primary curriculum content and the process for teaching it. The result could be an increased capacity for learning effective caring, which would provide a basis for nursing students to act ethically in response to human care problems and needs.

## References

Curtin, L., and M.J. Flaherty. 1982. *Nursing ethics: Theories and pragmatics.* Bowie, MD: Rovert J. Brady Co.

Davis, A. J., and M. A. Aroskar. (1983). *Ethical dilemmas and nursing practice.* East Norwalk, CT: Appleton-Century-Crofts.

Klein, R. 1963. *The self image of adult males in an Andean culture: A clinical exploration of a dynamic personality construct.* Ph.D. diss., New York University.

Leininger, M. 1981. *Caring: An essential human need.* Thorofare, NJ: Charles B. Slack. Reprint 1988 by Detroit: Wayne State University Press.

Leininger, M. 1984. *Care: The essence of nursing and health.* Thorofare, NJ: Charles B. Slack. Reprint 1988 by Detroit: Wayne State University Press.

Pearce, J., and S. Newton. 1963. *The conditions of human growth.* Secaucus, NJ: Citadel Press.

Ray, M. 1988. A philosophical analysis of caring within nursing. In *Caring: An essential human need.*, edited by M. Leininger, 25–36. Detroit: Wayne State University Press.

Stern, D. 1985. *The international world of the infant.* New York: Basic Books.

Sullivan, H. S. 1953. *The interpersonal theory of psychiatry.* New York: W. W. Norton.

Watson, J. 1979. *Nursing: The philosophy and science of caring.* Boston: Little, Brown.

Watson, J. 1981. Some issues related to the science of caring for nursing practice. In *Caring: An essential human need,* edited by M. Leininger, 61–67. Detroit: Wayne State University Press.

Watson, J. 1986. The Dean speaks out: Center for human caring established. *University of Colorado School for Nursing News,* December: 1, 6.

# Contributors

Anne J. Davis, R.N., Ph.D., F.A.A.N.
Professor of Nursing
College of Nursing
University of California
San Francisco, California

Sara T. Fry, R.N., Ph.D., F.A.A.N.
Associate Professor of Nursing
School of Nursing, University of
    Maryland
Baltimore, Maryland

Sally A. Gadow, R.N., Ph.D.
Associate Professor of Philosophy
The University of Texas
Institute for the Medical Humanities
Galveston, Texas

Brighid Kelly, R.N., M.S., Ph.D.
Associate Professor of Nursing
University of Cincinnati
College of Nursing and Health
Cincinnati, Ohio

Virginia Knowlden, R.N., M.A., Ed.D.
Associate Professor of Psychiatric-
    Mental Health Nursing
St. Joseph College
West Hartford, Connecticut

Madeleine M. Leininger, R.N., M.S.N.,
    Ph.D., L.H.D., D.S., F.A.A.N.,
    C.T.N.
Professor of Nursing, College of Nursing
Adjunct Professor of Anthropology,
    College of Liberal Arts
Wayne State University
Detroit, Michigan

Marilyn Miller, R.N., M.A.
Assistant Professor of Nursing
State University of New York
Health Science Center at Brooklyn
College of Nursing
Brooklyn, New York

Kathy Pike Parker, R.N., M.N.
Doctoral Candidate
Family and Community Nursing
School of Nursing
Georgia State University
Atlanta, Georgia

Phillis R. Schultz, R.N., Ph.D.
Professor of Nursing
College of Nursing
University of Colorado
Denver, Colorado

Robert C. Schultz, Ph.D.
Professor of Philosophy
University of Denver,
Denver, Colorado

Pamela Stinson Kidd, R.N., M.S.N.,
    Ph.D., C.E.N.
Assistant Professor of Nursing
University of Kentucky
College of Nursing
Lexington, Kentucky

Laura C. Zamora, R.N., M.A.
Assistant Professor of Nursing
State University of New York
Health Science Center at Brooklyn
College of Nursing
Brooklyn, New York

The manuscript was edited by Aimée Ergas. The book was designed by Elizabeth Hanson. The typeface for the text is Caledonia. The display faces are Caslon and Avant Garde.

Manufactured in the United States of America.